TABLE OF CONTENT

COPYRIGHT PAGE

Copyright © 2023

DEDICATION

This book is dedicated to all the brave individuals who have faced the challenges of a cancer diagnosis with unwavering strength, resilience, and courage. You are the true heroes in this journey.

To the healthcare professionals who provide compassionate care, the caregivers who offer unwavering support, and the friends and family who stand by their loved ones with love and understanding, your presence and dedication make a profound difference.

May this book serve as a beacon of hope, knowledge, and inspiration to those navigating the path of cancer, and may it offer guidance, comfort, and understanding to those who walk beside them.

INTRODUCTION

Welcome to "101 Tips for Living with Cancer." If you or someone you love has recently received a cancer diagnosis, you may be feeling a whirlwind of emotions: fear, confusion, uncertainty, and perhaps even a glimmer of hope. This journey is undeniably challenging, but it is also a testament to the strength, resilience, and courage that reside within each of us.

Cancer is not just a diagnosis; it's a life-altering event that touches every aspect of your existence. It can be a journey of unexpected twists and turns, triumphs and tribulations, and moments of profound self-discovery. It's a journey that can, at times, feel isolating, but it's also a journey shared by millions around the world who have faced or are facing similar challenges.

This book is not a medical textbook filled with complex jargon and treatment protocols. Instead, it is a compassionate companion that offers practical guidance, emotional support, and a wealth of insights to help you navigate the often-winding road of cancer. Within these pages, you'll find 101 tips designed to empower you, provide comfort, and promote well-being.

We'll explore topics ranging from understanding your diagnosis and treatment options to managing the physical and emotional symptoms that may arise. We'll delve into practical advice for everyday living, offer support for caregivers, and discuss the importance of building a strong support network.

Along the way, you'll discover stories of hope and inspiration from cancer survivors who have walked this path before you.

This book is not just about surviving cancer; it's about thriving despite the challenges it presents. It's about finding moments of joy, strength, and connection amidst the uncertainty. It's about making informed decisions, advocating for yourself, and embracing the life that continues to unfold, even in the face of adversity.

Whether you're a patient, a caregiver, a family member, or a friend, "101 Tips for Living with Cancer" is here to offer guidance, encouragement, and a reminder that you are not alone. Each tip is a small piece of a larger puzzle, a step along your unique journey. As you read through these pages, take what resonates with you, and leave behind what doesn't. Use this book as a resource to find answers, seek comfort, and spark inspiration.

Remember, your journey with cancer is as unique as you are, and this book is a supportive companion to help you navigate it with strength, dignity, and hope. You are not defined by your diagnosis, but by the courage and resilience with which you face it.

Together, we embark on a journey of healing, understanding, and empowerment. Let's take the first step on this path toward living with cancer, not just surviving it. Your journey is our journey, and we're here with you every step of the way.

With warmth and empathy,

CHAPTER ONE

UNDERSTANDING CANCER

Before we dive into the practical tips for living with cancer, it's essential to build a foundational understanding of what cancer is and how it affects the body. Knowledge is a powerful tool, and understanding your diagnosis is the first step toward making informed decisions about your care. In this section, we'll explore the fundamentals of cancer, its types, stages, and common misconceptions.

1.1 What Is Cancer

At its core, cancer is a group of diseases characterized by the uncontrolled growth and spread of abnormal cells in the body. These abnormal cells can form a mass or lump known as a tumor. However, not all tumors are cancerous; some are benign (non-cancerous) and do not pose a significant health threat.

Cancer can originate in almost any part of the body, from the skin to internal organs. The specific type of cancer is determined by the location and type of cells in which it begins. For example, breast cancer starts in the breast tissue, while lung cancer begins in the cells of the lung.

1.2 Types of Cancer

Cancer is not a single disease but a collection of different diseases, each with its characteristics and treatment approaches. Common types of cancer include:

- Breast Cancer
- Lung Cancer
- Colorectal Cancer
- Prostate Cancer
- Skin Cancer (Melanoma)
- Leukemia
- Lymphoma
- Pancreatic Cancer
- Ovarian Cancer
- Cervical Cancer

Each type of cancer has unique features, risk factors, and treatment options. Understanding the specific type of cancer, you have is crucial for tailoring your care plan.

1.3 Stages and Grading

Cancer is typically categorized into stages and grades to help healthcare professionals assess the extent of the disease and plan treatment. The stage of cancer refers to its size and whether it has spread to nearby lymph nodes or other parts of the body. Staging helps determine the best treatment approach.

Grading, on the other hand, assesses the appearance and behavior of cancer cells under a microscope. Grading can provide information about how quickly cancer is likely to grow and spread.

1.4 Common Misconceptions

Cancer is surrounded by a myriad of myths and misconceptions that can contribute to fear and misinformation. Some common misconceptions include:

- o **Cancer is always a death sentence:** While a cancer diagnosis is undoubtedly a serious matter, many people with cancer go on to live long and fulfilling lives, especially when diagnosed and treated early.
- o **Cancer is contagious:** Cancer is not contagious. You cannot "catch" cancer from someone else through physical contact.
- o **Cancer is solely caused by genetics:** While genetics can play a role in cancer risk, many factors, including lifestyle choices and environmental exposures, also contribute to the development of cancer.
- o **Alternative therapies can cure cancer:** While some alternative therapies can be complementary to conventional cancer treatments, they should not be used as a sole replacement for evidence-based treatments like surgery, radiation, or chemotherapy.

Understanding these fundamental aspects of cancer is the first step toward navigating your diagnosis with knowledge and confidence. In the subsequent tips, we'll delve deeper into various aspects of living with cancer, from treatment options to emotional well-being, so you can approach your journey with a comprehensive understanding.

CHAPTER TWO
COPING WITH DIAGNOSIS

2.1 Processing the News

Receiving a cancer diagnosis is an emotional and life-altering moment. It can feel like the ground beneath you has shifted, leaving you with a whirlwind of thoughts and emotions. In this section, we'll explore how to process the news of your diagnosis, cope with the initial shock, and take the first steps toward understanding and managing your journey.

The Initial Shock

It's entirely natural to experience a range of emotions when you first hear the words, "You have cancer." You might feel:

1. **Fear:** Fear of the unknown, fear of what lies ahead, fear of pain, and fear of the future.
2. **Anger:** Anger at the injustice of it all, anger at your body for "betraying" you, or anger at the world.
3. **Sadness:** A deep sense of grief, sadness for the life you thought you would have, or sadness for the people who love you.
4. **Denial:** A sense of disbelief, as if you're trapped in a surreal nightmare.
5. **Confusion:** An overwhelming sense of not knowing where to turn or what to do next.

All these emotions are valid and part of the process of coming to terms with your diagnosis. It's important to give yourself permission to feel whatever you're feeling. You don't have to have it all figured out right away.

Finding Support

Processing the news of a cancer diagnosis is not a journey you should undertake alone. Here's how you can seek support:

1. **Lean on Loved Ones:** Share the news with trusted family members and friends who can offer emotional support. They may not have all the answers, but their presence can be incredibly comforting.

2. **Ask Questions:** Reach out to your healthcare team and ask questions about your diagnosis, treatment options, and what to expect. Knowledge can empower you and reduce anxiety.

3. **Seek a Second Opinion:** If you have doubts or concerns about your diagnosis or treatment plan, consider seeking a second opinion from another healthcare provider. It's your right to ensure you're making the best decisions for your health.

4. **Explore Support Groups:** Consider joining a cancer support group, either in-person or online. Connecting with others who are going through similar experiences can provide valuable insights and a sense of belonging.

5. **Talk to a Therapist or Counselor:** A therapist or counselor experienced in cancer care can help you

process your emotions and develop coping strategies for the emotional challenges ahead.

Taking Care of Your Emotional Well-being

Your emotional well-being is just as important as your physical health during this time. Here are some tips for taking care of yourself:

1. **Practice Self-Compassion:** Be kind to yourself. This is a challenging journey, and you're doing your best.
2. **Stay Present:** Try to stay in the present moment rather than dwelling on the past or worrying about the future. Mindfulness techniques can help with this.
3. **Journal Your Thoughts:** Writing down your thoughts and emotions can be therapeutic. It can help you gain clarity and process your feelings.
4. **Create a Support Network:** Don't hesitate to reach out to friends, family, or support groups when you need to talk or simply be in the company of understanding individuals.
5. **Consider Professional Help:** If you find it challenging to cope with your emotions, consider seeking support from a mental health professional.

Remember, processing the news of your cancer diagnosis is a deeply personal journey. There's no "right" way to feel or react. Your emotions may ebb and flow, and that's okay. As you continue your journey, you'll discover inner strength and resilience you may not have known you possessed.

2.2 Building a Support System

One of the most crucial aspects of your journey with cancer is the support system you surround yourself with. The people who stand by your side—family, friends, healthcare professionals, and support groups—can provide emotional, practical, and invaluable support throughout your journey. In this section, we'll explore the importance of building a robust support system and offer guidance on how to do so.

Why a Support System Matters

A cancer diagnosis is a life-altering event that can be emotionally and physically overwhelming. Having a strong support system can make all the difference. Here's why it matters:

1. **Emotional Support:** Your support system can offer a listening ear, empathy, and a safe space to express your feelings and fears. They can provide comfort during difficult moments.

2. **Practical Assistance:** Whether it's helping with daily tasks, transportation to medical appointments, or managing household responsibilities, your support system can ease the burdens of daily life.

3. **Advocacy:** When navigating the healthcare system, having an advocate by your side can ensure that your voice is heard, questions are asked, and your preferences are respected.

4. **Information and Resources:** Your support system can help you gather information, research

treatment options, and connect you with valuable resources and support networks.

Who Can Be Part of Your Support System

Family and Friends: Loved ones can provide emotional support, accompany you to medical appointments, and help with day-to-day tasks.

1. **Healthcare Team:** Your doctors, nurses, and other healthcare professionals are a critical part of your support system. They provide medical expertise, guidance, and treatment options.
2. **Support Groups:** Consider joining a cancer support group, either in-person or online. These groups can provide a sense of community, shared experiences, and valuable insights.
3. **Mental Health Professionals**: Therapists, counselors, or psychologists with experience in cancer care can help you cope with the emotional challenges of your diagnosis.
4. **Advocacy Organizations:** Organizations dedicated to specific types of cancer often offer information, resources, and support services. They can connect you with others who have similar experiences.

Tips for Building and Nurturing Your Support System

1. **Communicate Your Needs:** Be open with your loved ones about what you need and how they can best support you. Clear communication is essential.

2. **Accept Help:** It's okay to accept assistance when it's offered. People genuinely want to help, so let them contribute in meaningful ways.

3. **Prioritize Self-Care:** Remember to take care of yourself, both physically and emotionally. You'll be better able to lean on your support system if you're feeling your best.

4. **Set Boundaries:** While support is essential, it's also important to set boundaries. Communicate when you need space or time alone.

5. **Express Gratitude:** Take the time to express gratitude to those who support you. A simple "thank you" can go a long way in nurturing these relationships.

6. **Stay Connected:** Maintain connections with friends and activities that bring you joy. Cancer is a part of your life, but it doesn't define your whole existence.

7. **Explore Professional Support:** If you're struggling emotionally, consider seeking help from a mental health professional with experience in cancer care.

Remember that your support system can evolve and change as your needs change throughout your cancer journey. The key is to surround yourself with individuals and resources that provide comfort, understanding, and strength. You're not alone on this path, and your support system is there to walk it with you.

2.3 Seeking Second Opinions

When it comes to a cancer diagnosis and treatment, the decisions you make are profoundly important. It's essential to gather as much information as possible and feel confident in your choices. Seeking a second opinion is a valuable step in this process, and in this section, we'll explore why it matters and how to go about it.

The Importance of Second Opinions

Receiving a cancer diagnosis is a momentous event, and the treatment decisions that follow can significantly impact your health and quality of life. Here's why seeking a second opinion is crucial:

1. **Confirmation:** A second opinion can confirm your initial diagnosis. While the accuracy of medical diagnoses is typically high, errors can occur. A second opinion can provide reassurance and confirm the path forward.

2. **Treatment Options:** Different oncologists may have varying approaches to treatment. A second opinion can help you explore alternative treatment options and make informed decisions about your care.

3. **Peace of Mind:** Seeking a second opinion can provide peace of mind, reduce anxiety, and increase your confidence in the chosen treatment plan.

4. **Clinical Trials:** Depending on your diagnosis, there may be clinical trials or experimental treatments available that you might not be aware of without seeking additional opinions.

When to Consider a Second Opinion

You might consider seeking a second opinion in the following situations:

1. **Complex or Rare Diagnoses:** If you have a complex or rare cancer diagnosis, getting multiple expert opinions can help ensure you're receiving the most accurate information and tailored treatment plan.

2. **Doubts or Uncertainty:** If you have doubts or uncertainties about your diagnosis or recommended treatment, it's a valid reason to seek a second opinion.

3. **Significant Treatment Decisions:** When faced with major treatment decisions, such as surgery or aggressive chemotherapy, a second opinion can provide valuable insights.

4. **Exploring All Options:** If you want to explore all available treatment options, including clinical trials or alternative therapies, a second opinion can help you make an informed choice.

How to Seek a Second Opinion

1. **Talk to Your Current Healthcare Team:** Start by discussing your intention to seek a second opinion with your current healthcare team. They should be supportive of your decision and may even help facilitate the process.

2. **Research Healthcare Providers:** Look for reputable cancer centers or specialists who have expertise in your specific type of cancer. Online resources, referrals from your current healthcare team, and recommendations from support groups can be valuable.

3. **Schedule an Appointment:** Contact the healthcare provider or cancer center you've chosen to schedule an appointment. Be prepared to provide your medical records, including test results, imaging, and pathology reports.

4. **Ask Questions:** During the second opinion appointment, ask questions about your diagnosis, treatment options, potential side effects, and prognosis. Be open about your concerns and preferences.

5. **Compare Opinions:** After obtaining a second opinion, compare the recommendations and insights you've received with those from your initial healthcare team. This process can help you make an informed decision about your care.

6. **Make Your Decision:** Ultimately, the decision about your treatment plan is yours to make. Consider all the information and recommendations carefully and choose the approach that aligns best with your goals and values.

Remember that seeking a second opinion is a common and respected practice in healthcare. It's not a sign of distrust; rather, it's a proactive step toward ensuring the best possible care for your unique situation.

Your health and well-being are paramount, and you deserve to have confidence in the decisions you make regarding your cancer treatment. Seeking second opinions is a powerful way to empower yourself in this journey.

2.4 Communicating with Loved Ones

One of the most challenging aspects of a cancer diagnosis is sharing the news with loved ones. It's natural to have concerns about how they will react and how to navigate these difficult conversations. In this section, we'll explore strategies for effective communication with family and friends as you embark on your cancer journey.

Opening the Conversation

Starting the conversation about your cancer diagnosis can be daunting, but it's an important step toward building a support system. Here's how to approach it:

1. **Choose the Right Time and Place:** Find a comfortable and quiet setting where you can talk without interruptions or distractions.
2. **Be Prepared:** Before the conversation, gather information about your diagnosis, treatment plan, and what to expect. Being informed will help you answer questions and provide reassurance.
3. **Share Honestly:** Be open and honest about your diagnosis. Avoid euphemisms or vague language that may lead to misunderstandings. Use clear and straightforward language.
4. **Express Your Feelings:** Share your own emotions and reactions to the diagnosis. This can help loved ones understand your perspective and provide emotional support.

5. **Encourage Questions:** Let your loved ones know that you're open to questions and that it's okay for them to express their concerns and feelings.

Managing Reactions

It's important to understand that your loved ones may have a range of emotional reactions to your diagnosis. These can include:

1. **Shock and Sadness:** Many people will initially react with shock, sadness, or even tears. They may need time to process the news.
2. **Concern:** Loved ones may express worry and concern for your well-being, which is a sign of their care and support.
3. **Guilt:** Some may experience feelings of guilt, thinking they could have done something to prevent your diagnosis or that they can't do enough to help.
4. **Fear:** Your diagnosis may trigger fears about losing you, which can be difficult for loved ones to cope with.

5. **Anger or Frustration:** Occasionally, people may respond with anger or frustration, not at you but at the unfairness of the situation.

Tips for Effective Communication

1. **Be Patient:** Recognize that reactions to your diagnosis may evolve over time. Be patient and understanding of your loved ones' emotional journeys.
2. **Encourage Openness:** Create an environment where your loved ones feel safe sharing their feelings and concerns with you. Listen actively and without judgment.
3. **Set Boundaries:** While it's important to be open, it's also crucial to set boundaries if certain conversations become too overwhelming or intrusive.
4. **Seek Support Together:** Encourage loved ones to seek their own support, whether through counseling, support groups, or talking to friends.
5. **Provide Resources:** Share information and resources about cancer and support services for both you and your loved ones. This can help them feel more equipped to navigate the journey with you.
6. **Celebrate Good Moments:** As you go through treatment and recovery, celebrate the positive moments and milestones with your loved ones. It can provide hope and motivation.

Maintaining Communication

Effective communication is an ongoing process. Continue to share updates on your health, treatment, and needs as your journey progresses. Regular, honest conversations can strengthen your relationships and provide a sense of connection during this challenging time.

Remember that your loved one's care deeply about your well-being, and they want to be there for you. By opening lines of communication and being patient and understanding, you can navigate your cancer journey together as a united front.

CHAPTER THREE
TREATMENT OPTIONS

3.1 Surgery, Radiation, and Chemotherapy

When it comes to treating cancer, there are several primary treatment modalities: surgery, radiation therapy, and chemotherapy. Each of these approaches plays a critical role in the fight against cancer. In this section, we'll delve into the basics of these treatments and what you can expect if they are part of your cancer journey.

Surgery: Removing the Cancer

Surgery is a common treatment for cancer, and its primary goal is to remove the tumor or cancerous tissue from the body. Here's what you need to know:

Types of Surgery: There are various surgical procedures used in cancer treatment, ranging from minimally invasive techniques to more extensive operations. The type of surgery you undergo depends on factors like the type and stage of cancer.

Preparation: Before surgery, your healthcare team will provide detailed instructions on how to prepare, including fasting and medication guidelines. You may also undergo preoperative tests.

The Procedure: During surgery, a skilled surgeon removes the cancerous tissue. Depending on the situation, surrounding healthy tissue and lymph nodes may also be removed to ensure that all cancer cells are eliminated.

Recovery: Recovery after surgery varies depending on the extent of the procedure. You'll receive postoperative care instructions and may need physical therapy or rehabilitation. Support from loved ones during this time is invaluable.

Radiation Therapy: Targeting Cancer Cells

Radiation therapy uses high-energy beams of radiation to target and destroy cancer cells. Here's what you should know:

1. **Types of Radiation:** There are different types of radiation therapy, including external beam radiation (where the radiation source is outside the body) and internal radiation (where radiation is delivered directly to the tumor, also known as brachytherapy).

2. **Treatment Sessions:** Radiation therapy is typically administered in multiple sessions over several weeks. The exact schedule and duration depend on your specific treatment plan.

3. **Side Effects:** Radiation therapy may cause side effects, such as fatigue, skin changes, and localized discomfort. Your healthcare team will monitor your progress and help manage any side effects.

4. **Precision and Planning:** Radiation therapy is highly precise, with the goal of targeting cancer cells

while sparing healthy tissue as much as possible. Advanced imaging and planning techniques ensure accuracy.

Chemotherapy: Systemic Treatment

Chemotherapy is a systemic treatment that uses drugs to target and destroy cancer cells throughout the body. Here's what you should be aware of:

1. **Administration:** Chemotherapy can be administered orally in pill form or intravenously through a vein. The choice of chemotherapy drugs and the schedule depend on the type and stage of cancer.
2. **Side Effects:** Chemotherapy can have side effects, including nausea, fatigue, hair loss, and changes in blood cell counts. Supportive care measures can help manage these side effects.
3. **Combination Therapies:** In some cases, chemotherapy is used in combination with other treatments, such as radiation.

3.2 Immunotherapy and Targeted Therapies

In the ever-evolving landscape of cancer treatment, two remarkable advancements have emerged: immunotherapy and targeted therapies. These innovative approaches are changing the way we combat cancer, offering new hope and possibilities. In this section, we'll explore the fundamentals of immunotherapy and targeted therapies, and how they can be integral to your cancer journey.

Immunotherapy: Empowering Your Immune System

Immunotherapy is a groundbreaking treatment that harnesses the body's own immune system to fight cancer. Here's what you need to know:

1. **How It Works:** Immunotherapy boosts your immune system's ability to recognize and attack cancer cells. It can activate immune cells or block signals that cancer cells use to evade detection.

2. **Types of Immunotherapy:** There are different types of immunotherapy, including checkpoint inhibitors, cancer vaccines, and adoptive cell therapy. The specific type depends on your cancer and its characteristics.

3. **Treatment Schedule:** Immunotherapy is typically administered through intravenous (IV) infusions or injections. Treatment schedules vary, and you'll work

closely with your healthcare team to determine the best approach.

4. **Side Effects:** While immunotherapy generally has fewer side effects than traditional treatments like chemotherapy, it can still cause immune-related side effects. These may include fatigue, skin rashes, and inflammation of the digestive tract. It's essential to communicate any symptoms with your healthcare team.

5. **Response and Durability:** Immunotherapy can lead to durable responses, meaning that the benefits can last for an extended period, even after treatment is completed.

Targeted Therapies: Precision Medicine

Targeted therapies are a class of cancer treatments that focus on specific molecules or pathways involved in the growth and spread of cancer cells. Here's what you should know:

1. **Targeted Molecules:** These therapies are designed to "target" particular molecules or proteins that are involved in the development and progression of cancer. By doing so, they interfere with the cancer's ability to grow and divide.

2. **Personalized Treatment:** Targeted therapies are often personalized based on the specific genetic and molecular characteristics of your cancer. This allows for a more precise and effective approach.

3. **Administration:** Targeted therapies are typically taken orally in pill form, making them more convenient than traditional chemotherapy.
4. **Side Effects:** Like all treatments, targeted therapies can have side effects, which vary depending on the drug. Common side effects may include skin rash, diarrhea, and hypertension. Your healthcare team will closely monitor your progress.
5. **Combination Therapy:** In some cases, targeted therapies may be used in combination with other treatments, such as chemotherapy or radiation therapy, to maximize their effectiveness.

The Promise of Precision and Empowerment

Immunotherapy and targeted therapies represent a new era in cancer treatment. They offer the promise of more precise and less toxic treatments, with the potential for improved outcomes and quality of life.

It's important to remember that not all cancers respond to these therapies, and their effectiveness can vary from person to person. Your healthcare team will work with you to determine if these treatments are suitable for your specific cancer type and stage.

While these therapies hold great promise, it's essential to approach them with realistic expectations and a thorough understanding of your treatment plan. Together with your healthcare team, you can explore the possibilities of immunotherapy and targeted therapies as part of your cancer journey.

3.3 Complementary and Alternative Medicine

In addition to conventional cancer treatments, many individuals explore complementary and alternative medicine (CAM) to enhance their overall well-being and manage the side effects of cancer and its treatments. While these approaches should always be discussed with your healthcare team, this section will provide an overview of CAM and how it can complement your cancer journey.

Understanding Complementary and Alternative Medicine

Complementary and alternative medicine encompasses a wide range of therapies and practices that are used alongside or instead of conventional medical treatments. Here are some key points to consider:

1. **Complementary vs. Alternative:** "Complementary" therapies are used alongside conventional treatments to enhance their effectiveness or manage side effects. "Alternative" therapies are used instead of conventional treatments. It's crucial to differentiate between the two.

2. **Holistic Approach:** CAM often takes a holistic approach, addressing not only the physical aspects of cancer but also the emotional, mental, and spiritual dimensions.

3. **Types of CAM:** CAM includes practices such as acupuncture, massage therapy, yoga, meditation,

dietary supplements, herbal remedies, and mind-body techniques, among others.

Benefits and Considerations

When exploring CAM, it's essential to be informed and consult with your healthcare team. Here are some benefits and considerations to keep in mind:

1. **Symptom Management:** CAM can help manage common cancer-related symptoms such as pain, nausea, fatigue, and anxiety. Techniques like acupuncture and massage therapy can provide relief.
2. **Enhanced Well-being:** Many people find that CAM therapies improve their overall well-being, reduce stress, and enhance their quality of life during and after cancer treatment.
3. **Safety and Research:** It's crucial to use CAM therapies safely and be aware of potential interactions with conventional treatments. Not all CAM therapies are supported by rigorous scientific research, so consult your healthcare team for guidance.
4. **Open Communication:** Always inform your healthcare team about any CAM therapies you're considering. They can provide insights into potential benefits, risks, and compatibility with your treatment plan.

Integrating CAM into Your Cancer Journey

If you're interested in exploring CAM therapies, here are some steps to consider:

Consult Your Healthcare Team: Talk to your oncologist or healthcare provider about your interest in CAM. They can help you evaluate which therapies may be safe and beneficial for your specific situation.

1. **Research and Choose Wisely:** Look for reputable sources of information on CAM and consider seeking referrals to CAM practitioners with experience in cancer care.
2. **Safety First:** Always prioritize safety. Discuss potential CAM therapies and supplements with your healthcare team to ensure they won't interfere with your conventional treatments.
3. **Mind-Body Practices:** Mindfulness, meditation, and yoga are examples of mind-body practices that can promote relaxation and emotional well-being.
4. **Nutritional Support:** Consult a registered dietitian with expertise in oncology nutrition to discuss dietary changes, supplements, and nutrition strategies that support your health.
5. **Supportive Therapies:** Consider therapies such as acupuncture, massage, and music therapy, which can alleviate side effects and enhance your comfort.

Remember that the integration of CAM should complement and enhance your conventional treatment plan, not replace it. Your healthcare team is your primary source of guidance and should be involved in all decisions related to your care.

3.4 Clinical Trials

Clinical trials are at the forefront of advancing cancer treatment and care. They offer the promise of groundbreaking discoveries and innovative therapies. In this section, we'll explore the significance of clinical trials, their potential benefits, and how you can navigate this avenue as part of your cancer journey.

What Are Clinical Trials

Clinical trials are research studies designed to evaluate the safety and effectiveness of new treatments, therapies, or interventions. They are conducted with human participants and are an essential step in the development of new medical advancements. Here's what you should know:

1. **Phases of Clinical Trials:** Clinical trials are typically conducted in phases. Phase I trials focus on safety and dosage, Phase II trials assess effectiveness and side effects, and Phase III trials compare the new treatment to standard treatments.

2. **Informed Consent:** Before enrolling in a clinical trial, you will receive detailed information about the study's purpose, procedures, potential risks, and benefits. You must provide informed consent before participating.

3. **Diverse Participants:** Clinical trials involve participants from various backgrounds and with different types and stages of cancer. This diversity is critical for assessing how treatments work in different populations.

Potential Benefits of Clinical Trials

Participating in a clinical trial offers several potential benefits:

Access to Cutting-Edge Treatments: Clinical trials often provide access to therapies that are not yet available to the public. This can be especially valuable if standard treatments are not effective for your condition.

1. **Contributing to Research:** By participating, you contribute to the advancement of medical knowledge and may help future cancer patients benefit from improved treatments.
2. **Close Monitoring:** Participants in clinical trials receive close monitoring and medical care from a dedicated healthcare team, which can enhance your overall care.
3. **Personalized Approach:** Clinical trials may offer treatments that are tailored to your specific cancer type and genetic profile.

Navigating Clinical Trials

If you're interested in exploring clinical trials, here are steps to consider:

1. **Discuss with Your Healthcare Team:** Talk to your oncologist or healthcare provider about the possibility of participating in a clinical trial. They can

assess whether you meet the eligibility criteria and discuss potential trials that align with your needs.

2. **Ask Questions:** Don't hesitate to ask questions about the trial, including its purpose, treatment details, potential risks, and expected outcomes. Understanding the trial is essential for making an informed decision.

3. **Consider Your Goals:** Reflect on your goals and priorities. Are you seeking a new treatment option, or are you comfortable with your current care plan? Clinical trials are voluntary, and your preferences should guide your decision.

4. **Review Informed Consent:** Carefully review the informed consent document provided by the trial investigators. Seek clarification on any uncertainties before signing.

5. **Support and Advocacy:** Consider involving a trusted loved one or advocate in your decision-making process. They can help you gather information and provide emotional support.

6. **Regular Updates:** If you decide to participate in a clinical trial, maintain open communication with your healthcare team. They will provide updates on your progress and treatment plan.

The Hope and Potential of Clinical Trials

Clinical trials are a testament to the resilience and determination of the medical community in the fight against cancer. They offer hope for improved treatments and, ultimately, a future where cancer is more effectively managed and even cured.

Whether or not you choose to participate in a clinical trial, your decision should be based on your unique circumstances, values, and goals. Your healthcare team is your most valuable resource for guiding you through this complex and potentially life-changing process.

CHAPTER FOUR
MANAGING SYMTOMS

4.1 Nausea and Fatigue

Nausea and fatigue are common side effects of cancer and its treatments, but there are strategies to help you cope and improve your quality of life. In this section, we'll explore how to manage nausea and fatigue effectively, allowing you to better navigate your cancer journey.

Nausea: Taming the Queasiness

Nausea is a sensation of queasiness or an upset stomach, which can be a distressing symptom during cancer treatment. Here's what you need to know:

1. **Causes:** Nausea can result from chemotherapy, radiation therapy, surgery, or medications. It may also be triggered by anxiety or changes in your diet.
2. **Preventive Medications:** Your healthcare team may prescribe anti-nausea medications to prevent or alleviate nausea associated with cancer treatment. It's essential to take these medications as directed.
3. **Dietary Adjustments:** Avoid heavy or greasy meals before treatment. opt for small, frequent meals and bland foods like crackers, toast, and ginger tea, which can help soothe your stomach.
4. **Hydration:** Staying hydrated is crucial. Sip water or clear fluids throughout the day to prevent dehydration,

but avoid drinking large amounts in one go, as this can trigger nausea.

5. **Ginger:** Ginger has natural anti-nausea properties. Consider ginger candies, tea, or supplements to ease nausea.

6. **Acupressure Bands:** Some individuals find relief from nausea by wearing acupressure bands, which apply gentle pressure to specific wrist points.

Fatigue: Managing the Overwhelming Tiredness

Fatigue is extreme tiredness or weakness that can impact your daily activities and quality of life. Coping with cancer-related fatigue is essential for maintaining your well-being:

1. **Physical Activity:** Engage in light physical activity, such as walking or gentle stretching, to maintain muscle strength and energy levels. Consult with your healthcare team about the right level of activity for your condition.

2. **Rest and Sleep:** Prioritize adequate rest and sleep. Establish a regular sleep routine, practice relaxation techniques, and create a comfortable sleep environment.

3. **Nutrition:** A balanced diet can help combat fatigue. Eat a variety of nutrient-rich foods and consider consulting a registered dietitian with expertise in oncology nutrition.

4. **Energy Conservation:** Plan your day to conserve energy. Break tasks into smaller, manageable segments

and prioritize essential activities. Don't hesitate to ask for help with tasks when needed.

5. **Mind-Body Practices:** Practices like meditation, mindfulness, and deep breathing exercises can help manage stress and fatigue. Consider incorporating these into your daily routine.

6. **Emotional Support:** Share your feelings of fatigue with your loved ones and healthcare team. They can offer emotional support and help you manage your energy levels.

Open Communication with Your Healthcare Team

Nausea and fatigue are side effects that can vary in severity from person to person. Open communication with your healthcare team is crucial:

1. **Report Symptoms:** Inform your healthcare team about your nausea and fatigue symptoms. They can adjust your treatment plan or provide additional support.

2. **Medication Management:** If anti-nausea medications aren't effective, your healthcare team can explore alternative options or adjust the dosage.

3. **Fatigue Assessment:** Discuss your fatigue levels during medical appointments. Your healthcare team can assess whether there are underlying causes that require attention.

Remember that you're not alone in managing these symptoms. Many cancer patients experience nausea and fatigue, and there are effective strategies and treatments available to help you cope. By actively addressing these challenges, you can improve your overall quality of life during your cancer journey.

4.2 Pain Management

Pain is a common symptom experienced by individuals living with cancer, but it can be effectively managed, allowing you to enhance your quality of life and better cope with the challenges of your cancer journey. In this section, we'll explore various aspects of pain management and strategies to help you find relief.

Understanding Cancer Pain

Cancer-related pain can result from various factors, including the tumor pressing on nerves or organs, cancer treatments, or the side effects of medications. Here's what you need to know:

1. **Types of Pain:** Cancer pain can be categorized as acute (short-term) or chronic (long-term). It may be localized, such as at the tumor site, or more generalized.
2. **Assessment:** Effective pain management begins with a thorough assessment by your healthcare team. They will ask you about the location, intensity, and character of your pain, as well as its impact on your daily life.
3. **Pain Scale:** Healthcare providers often use a pain scale (usually from 0 to 10) to help assess and track your pain levels. This scale helps determine the effectiveness of pain management strategies.

Multimodal Approach to Pain Management

Pain management is most effective when approached from multiple angles. Consider the following strategies:

1. **Medications:** Your healthcare team may prescribe medications to manage pain. These can include opioids, non-opioid pain relievers, and adjuvant medications that target specific types of pain.
2. **Pain Diary:** Keeping a pain diary can help you track when pain occurs, its severity, and any triggers. This information is valuable for your healthcare team in adjusting your pain management plan.
3. **Non-Pharmacological Techniques:** Non-pharmacological approaches like physical therapy, acupuncture, massage, and relaxation techniques can complement medication-based pain management.
4. **Mind-Body Practices:** Practices such as mindfulness meditation and deep breathing exercises can help you cope with pain and reduce stress, which can exacerbate discomfort.
5. **Nutrition and Hydration:** Proper nutrition and hydration are essential for overall well-being and can indirectly impact your pain levels.

Open Communication with Your Healthcare Team

Effective pain management requires open communication with your healthcare team:

1. **Regular Updates:** Inform your healthcare team about any changes in your pain levels. Regular communication helps them adjust your pain management plan as needed.

2. **Medication Management:** If you're prescribed pain medications, follow the dosing instructions carefully. Report any side effects or concerns to your healthcare provider.

3. **Adjustments:** Be prepared for adjustments to your pain management plan as your condition changes. Your healthcare team will work with you to find the most effective approach.

4. **Quality of Life:** Discuss your goals and priorities with your healthcare team. Pain management should align with your desire to maintain a good quality of life.

Advocacy and Self-Care

As you navigate pain management, remember that you are your best advocate:

1. **Speak Up:** Don't hesitate to voice your concerns, preferences, and questions about pain management. Your healthcare team is there to support you.

2. **Self-Care:** Incorporate self-care practices into your routine. This can include maintaining a healthy lifestyle, seeking emotional support, and engaging in activities that bring you joy and relaxation.

3. **Support System:** Lean on your support system—family, friends, and support groups—during challenging times. They can provide emotional support and practical assistance.

Managing cancer-related pain is a crucial aspect of your journey, and finding effective strategies can significantly improve your well-being. Remember that you don't have to face pain alone, and your healthcare team is here to guide you toward relief and comfort.

4.3 Hair Loss and Skin Changes

Cancer and its treatments can bring about physical changes to your body, including hair loss and skin changes. These alterations, while challenging, can be managed, and this section aims to provide you with guidance on coping with these changes and maintaining your self-esteem during your cancer journey.

Hair Loss: Embracing Your Inner Beauty

Hair loss, known medically as alopecia, can be emotionally distressing for many cancer patients. Here's how to navigate this aspect of your journey:

1. **Understanding Causes:** Hair loss can result from chemotherapy, radiation therapy, immunotherapy, or targeted therapies. It's typically temporary and reversible.

2. **Consider Hair Options:** You may choose to explore wigs, scarves, hats, or hairpieces as alternatives during hair loss. Some individuals prefer to embrace their natural appearance.

3. **Scalp Care:** Be gentle with your scalp during hair loss. Use mild, sulfate-free shampoos and avoid excessive heat when showering.

4. **Sun Protection:** If your scalp is exposed, protect it from the sun by wearing a hat or applying sunscreen with a high SPF rating.

5. **Support Groups:** Joining a cancer support group can provide emotional support and connect you with others who have experienced hair loss.

6. **Embrace Change:** Remember that hair loss is a temporary aspect of your cancer journey. As your treatments conclude, your hair will typically start to grow back.

Skin Changes: Nurturing Your Skin

Cancer treatments can cause various skin changes, including dryness, sensitivity, and increased vulnerability to sun damage. Here's how to care for your skin:

1. **Hydration:** Keep your skin well-hydrated by applying fragrance-free moisturizers regularly. Avoid hot showers and opt for lukewarm water.

2. **Gentle Cleansing:** Use mild, unscented cleansers and avoid harsh scrubs or exfoliants that can irritate your skin.

3. **Sun Protection:** Protect your skin from the sun's harmful UV rays. Use sunscreen with a high SPF rating and wear protective clothing when outdoors.

4. **Avoid Irritants:** Avoid using perfumes, harsh detergents, and products containing alcohol, which can further irritate sensitive skin.

5. **Consult a Dermatologist:** If you experience severe skin issues, consult a dermatologist with experience in cancer care. They can provide specialized guidance and treatment recommendations.

Self-Care and Self-Expression

Maintaining self-esteem and a sense of self-expression during cancer-related physical changes is essential:

1. **Self-Care Rituals:** Create a self-care routine that includes gentle skincare, relaxation techniques, and activities that bring you joy.
2. **Express Yourself:** Embrace your individuality. Whether you choose to wear a headscarf, a colorful hat, or confidently showcase your bald head, remember that your appearance is just one facet of your identity.
3. **Supportive Network:** Surround yourself with a supportive network of loved ones who appreciate your inner beauty and strength.
4. **Confidence Building:** Focus on your strengths, talents, and accomplishments. Your beauty radiates from within, and your journey is a testament to your resilience.

Embracing Your Authentic Self

While cancer and its treatments may bring about changes to your physical appearance, they cannot diminish your inner strength, resilience, and beauty. Embrace your authentic self, love yourself through these changes, and remember that you are a remarkable individual on a unique journey of healing and self-discovery.

4.4 Nutrition and Appetite

Maintaining good nutrition during your cancer journey is crucial for your overall well-being, energy levels, and treatment outcomes. However, cancer and its treatments can often impact your appetite and dietary habits. In this section, we'll explore strategies to support your nutrition and appetite as you navigate this challenging time.

The Importance of Nutrition

Proper nutrition plays a pivotal role in your cancer journey:

1. **Energy and Strength:** Adequate nutrition provides the energy and nutrients your body needs to cope with the demands of cancer treatments and maintain muscle strength.
2. **Immune Function:** A well-balanced diet can bolster your immune system, helping your body fight infections and recover more effectively.
3. **Tolerance to Treatment:** Good nutrition can improve your tolerance to cancer treatments, potentially reducing the risk of treatment interruptions.
4. **Quality of Life:** A nutritious diet can enhance your overall quality of life, manage side effects, and support emotional well-being.

Managing Appetite Changes

Cancer and its treatments can bring about changes in your appetite, taste preferences, and digestion. Here are some strategies to help:

1. **Small, Frequent Meals:** Instead of three large meals, consider eating smaller, more frequent meals throughout the day. This can be less overwhelming and help maintain your energy levels.
2. **Nutrient-Dense Foods:** Focus on nutrient-dense foods that provide essential vitamins and minerals. These include fruits, vegetables, whole grains, lean proteins, and healthy fats.
3. **Stay Hydrated:** Adequate hydration is essential. Sip water, herbal teas, or clear broths throughout the day to prevent dehydration.
4. **Flavor Enhancement:** Experiment with herbs and spices to add flavor to your meals. Tangy or tart flavors can sometimes be more appealing.
5. **Texture Modifications:** If certain textures are unappealing due to treatment side effects, consider blending or pureeing foods to make them more palatable.
6. **Consult a Dietitian:** A registered dietitian with expertise in oncology nutrition can provide personalized guidance, meal plans, and tips tailored to your specific needs.

Special Dietary Considerations

Your dietary needs may vary depending on your cancer type, treatment, and any side effects you're experiencing. Here are some considerations:

1. **High-Protein Diet:** If you're losing weight or muscle mass, a high-protein diet may be beneficial to help you maintain strength.
2. **Dietary Restrictions:** Some treatments may require specific dietary restrictions. Consult with your healthcare team or dietitian for guidance.
3. **Supplements:** In certain cases, your healthcare team may recommend dietary supplements to address nutritional deficiencies.

Emotional and Social Support

Eating can be an emotional and social experience, and it's essential to consider the emotional aspect of nutrition:

1. **Emotional Support:** Seek emotional support from loved ones, support groups, or counseling if you're struggling with dietary changes or appetite issues.
2. **Social Connection:** Sharing meals with loved ones can be a source of comfort and joy. Even if your appetite is diminished, the social aspect of dining together can be valuable.

Patient and Empowered Choices

Remember that you are in control of your nutrition journey:

1. **Advocacy:** Advocate for your dietary preferences and needs with your healthcare team and loved ones.
2. **Flexibility:** Be open to trying new foods and approaches. What works for one person may not work for another, so be flexible in finding what suits you best.
3. **Patience:** Your appetite and taste preferences may change over time. Be patient with yourself as you adapt to these changes.

Nutrition and appetite are integral components of your cancer journey. By making informed choices, seeking support, and prioritizing your nutritional needs, you can help optimize your health and well-being as you navigate this challenging path.

5.1 Dealing with Fear and Anxiety

A cancer diagnosis often brings about fear and anxiety, which can be overwhelming. In this section, we'll explore strategies to help you cope with these challenging emotions, allowing you to find strength and resilience during your cancer journey.

Understanding Fear and Anxiety

It's natural to experience fear and anxiety when facing cancer:

1. **Fear of the Unknown:** The uncertainty that comes with a cancer diagnosis can be frightening. You may worry about the future, treatment outcomes, and what lies ahead.
2. **Treatment Anxiety:** Cancer treatments can be physically and emotionally taxing. Fear of side effects, pain, and treatment efficacy is common.
3. **Emotional Impact:** The emotional toll of cancer, including fear of death, changes in body image, and concern about the impact on loved ones, can lead to anxiety.
4. **Social Isolation:** Feelings of isolation and alienation may arise, as you grapple with the emotional weight of cancer.

Coping Strategies for Fear and Anxiety

Coping with fear and anxiety is essential for your well-being and peace of mind. Here are strategies to help you manage these emotions:

1. **Open Communication:** Share your fears and concerns with your healthcare team, loved ones, or a counselor. Expressing your feelings can alleviate some of the emotional burden.

2. **Mindfulness and Relaxation:** Practice mindfulness meditation, deep breathing exercises, or progressive muscle relaxation to calm your mind and reduce anxiety.

3. **Support Groups:** Joining a cancer support group can provide a sense of community and connection with others who understand what you're going through.

4. **Seek Professional Help:** If anxiety becomes overwhelming and interferes with your daily life, consider seeking support from a mental health professional who specializes in cancer-related issues.

5. **Educate Yourself:** Knowledge can be empowering. Learning about your cancer type, treatment options, and expected side effects can demystify the process and reduce anxiety.

6. **Set Realistic Goals:** Focus on attainable goals and milestones in your cancer journey. Breaking your journey into smaller steps can make it feel more manageable.

Managing Anxiety During Treatment

During cancer treatment, anxiety may intensify due to various stressors. Here are strategies to manage anxiety during this phase:

1. **Distraction Techniques:** Engage in activities that provide a mental escape from cancer-related thoughts. Reading, watching movies, or pursuing hobbies can be helpful distractions.
2. **Physical Activity:** Incorporate gentle physical activity into your routine, if possible. Exercise releases endorphins, which can improve your mood and reduce anxiety.
3. **Medication and Counseling:** Consult your healthcare team about medications or counseling services that can help manage anxiety during treatment.
4. **Self-Compassion:** Be kind to yourself and recognize that it's okay to have moments of fear and anxiety. Self-compassion is an essential part of emotional well-being.

A Journey of Resilience

Your cancer journey is a testament to your resilience and strength. Remember that it's normal to experience fear and anxiety, but you have the capacity to cope and thrive:

1. **Positive Affirmations:** Repeat positive affirmations daily to boost your self-esteem and sense of control.

2. **Visualization:** Practice visualization techniques, where you imagine yourself successfully navigating your cancer journey.

3. **Focus on the Present:** Ground yourself in the present moment to alleviate worries about the past or future. Mindfulness techniques can help with this.

Embracing Support and Self-Care

Seeking support and prioritizing self-care are essential components of coping with fear and anxiety:

1. **Support Network:** Lean on your support network of loved ones, friends, and healthcare providers. They are there to help you through this journey.
2. **Self-Care Rituals:** Create a self-care routine that nurtures your physical, emotional, and spiritual well-being.
3. **Hope and Resilience:** Hold onto hope and recognize your inner resilience. Your journey may be challenging, but you have the inner strength to persevere.

Moving Forward with Courage

Fear and anxiety are natural responses to a cancer diagnosis, but they need not define your journey. By embracing support, practicing self-care, and using coping strategies, you can move forward with courage and resilience, facing each day with determination and hope.

5.2 Coping with Depression

Cancer can bring about a range of emotions, including depression. While it's normal to experience moments of sadness and grief during your cancer journey, persistent and overwhelming feelings of depression can be challenging. In this section, we'll explore strategies to help you cope with depression and find a sense of hope and resilience.

Understanding Depression

Depression is a complex emotional state that can affect anyone, including cancer patients:

1. **Persistent Sadness:** Depression often manifests as persistent feelings of sadness, hopelessness, and despair.
2. **Physical Symptoms**: It can be accompanied by physical symptoms such as fatigue, changes in appetite and sleep patterns, and a lack of interest in activities you once enjoyed.
3. **Impact on Daily Life:** Depression can interfere with your ability to concentrate, make decisions, and carry out daily tasks.
4. **Isolation:** Feelings of isolation and withdrawal from social activities are common in depression.

Recognizing Depression

Recognizing and acknowledging depression is the first step toward coping with it:

1. **Symptom Awareness:** Be aware of common symptoms of depression, including feelings of sadness, changes in sleep and appetite, fatigue, and loss of interest in activities.

2. **Open Communication:** Share your feelings with a trusted loved one, a support group, or a mental health professional. Talking about your emotions can be therapeutic.

3. **Consult Your Healthcare Team:** Inform your healthcare team about your emotional state. They can provide guidance on managing depression as part of your cancer care plan.

Coping Strategies for Depression

Coping with depression is a multifaceted journey. Here are strategies to help you navigate this emotional terrain:

1. **Psychotherapy:** Consider individual or group therapy with a mental health professional experienced in cancer-related depression.
2. **Medication:** In some cases, medication may be prescribed to help manage depression. Discuss this option with your healthcare team.
3. **Support Network:** Lean on your support network of friends and family. Don't hesitate to ask for assistance or emotional support when needed.
4. **Self-Care Rituals:** Prioritize self-care practices, including relaxation techniques, physical activity, and mindfulness meditation.
5. **Creative Expression:** Engage in creative outlets such as art, writing, or music to channel your emotions and find moments of joy.
6. **Setting Realistic Goals:** Break tasks into manageable steps and set realistic goals to regain a sense of accomplishment.
7. **Support Groups:** Consider joining a cancer support group where you can connect with others who may be experiencing similar emotions.

The Power of Self-Compassion

Self-compassion is a vital component of coping with depression:

1. **Acceptance:** Accept that experiencing depression is not a sign of weakness. It's a natural response to the challenges you're facing.

2. **Self-Love:** Treat yourself with the same kindness and understanding that you would offer to a loved one in a similar situation.

3. **Patience:** Be patient with yourself as you navigate depression. Healing takes time, and each day brings the opportunity for progress.

Embracing Hope and Resilience

Depression may be a part of your cancer journey, but it need not define it. By seeking support, practicing self-care, and using coping strategies, you can find moments of hope and resilience:

1. **Hope:** Hold onto hope, even in the darkest moments. Your journey may be challenging, but there is always the potential for brighter days ahead.
2. **Resilience:** Recognize your inner strength and resilience. You have the capacity to overcome depression and emerge from this experience stronger.
3. **Moving Forward:** Focus on taking one step at a time, one day at a time. Each small step is a testament to your courage and determination.

You Are Not Alone

Remember that you are not alone in your struggle with depression. Many cancer patients experience this emotional challenge, and there is help and support available. Your journey is unique, and by seeking assistance and nurturing your well-being, you can find the strength to cope with depression and move forward with resilience.

5.3 Finding Joy and Laughter

Amid the challenges of a cancer diagnosis and treatment, it's important to remember that joy and laughter can be powerful allies in your journey. In this section, we'll explore how to seek moments of joy, embrace laughter, and infuse your life with positivity during this trying time.

The Healing Power of Joy

Joy is a profound emotion that can uplift your spirits, enhance your overall well-being, and provide strength during challenging moments:

1. **Emotional Resilience:** Experiencing joy can boost your emotional resilience and help you navigate difficult emotions more effectively.
2. **Stress Reduction:** Laughter and joy trigger the release of endorphins, your body's natural feel-good chemicals, which can reduce stress and pain.
3. **Enhanced Immunity:** A positive outlook and joyful moments may support your immune system, contributing to your overall health.

Seeking Moments of Joy

Cultivating joy involves actively seeking out experiences and activities that bring happiness to your life:

1. **Gratitude Practice:** Start each day by reflecting on the things you're grateful for. This practice can shift your perspective toward positivity.

2. **Hobbies and Passions:** Engage in activities you love or explore new hobbies that spark your interest. Creativity and self-expression can bring immense joy.

3. **Nature Connection:** Spend time in nature, whether it's a peaceful walk in the park, listening to birdsong, or watching a beautiful sunset.

4. **Laughter Yoga:** Consider joining a laughter yoga group or practice laughter exercises at home. Laughter is contagious and can be therapeutic.

5. **Connect with Loved Ones:** Surround yourself with supportive loved ones who bring joy and laughter into your life.

Embracing Laughter

Laughter is a universal language of joy, and it can be a valuable tool in your cancer journey:

1. **Laughter as Medicine:** Studies have shown that laughter can improve mood, reduce stress, and even have physical health benefits.
2. **Comedy and Entertainment:** Watch comedies, read humorous books, or attend live comedy shows. Laughter derived from entertainment can be a powerful mood booster.
3. **Social Laughter:** Share moments of laughter with friends and family. Laughter can strengthen bonds and provide mutual support.
4. **Laugh at Yourself:** Don't be afraid to laugh at your own quirks and mishaps. A sense of humor about life's imperfections can be liberating.

Positive Mindset and Resilience

A positive mindset and resilience can go hand in hand with finding joy and laughter:

1. **Coping Mechanism:** Embracing joy and humor can be a valuable coping mechanism during challenging times.
2. **Resilience:** Resilience is the ability to bounce back from adversity. Cultivating joy and laughter can enhance your resilience.

3. **Mind-Body Connection:** Positive emotions and laughter can have a beneficial impact on your overall health, potentially improving your response to treatments.

Joy in Everyday Moments

Remember that joy can be found in the simplest of moments:

1. **Smiles:** Share smiles with others, whether it's with a stranger, a healthcare provider, or a loved one. Smiles are contagious and can brighten someone's day.
2. **Mindfulness:** Practice mindfulness to savor the present moment. Even ordinary moments can be filled with beauty and joy when viewed mindfully.
3. **Celebrations:** Celebrate milestones, no matter how small. Each step forward in your cancer journey is worth acknowledging and celebrating.

Your Journey, Your Joy

Your cancer journey is uniquely yours, and finding joy and laughter can be an integral part of it:

1. **Personalized Approach:** Discover what brings you joy and tailor your activities to your preferences. Your journey to joy is personal and unique.
2. **Self-Compassion:** Be kind to yourself and recognize that it's okay to experience moments of joy, even amid challenges.
3. **Shared Joy:** Share your moments of joy and laughter with others. Your positivity can inspire and uplift those around you.

A Reminder of Resilience

Amid the trials of cancer, finding joy and laughter is a testament to your resilience and strength. These moments remind you of your ability to embrace life's beauty and overcome adversity, one joyful moment at a time.

5.4 Mindfulness and Meditation

Amid the challenges that cancer presents, the practices of mindfulness and meditation offer powerful tools for calming the mind, reducing stress, and finding moments of peace and clarity. In this section, we'll explore how mindfulness and meditation can be valuable companions on your cancer journey.

Understanding Mindfulness and Meditation

Mindfulness is the practice of being fully present in the moment, without judgment. Meditation is a specific technique used to cultivate mindfulness. Here's how they can benefit you:

1. **Stress Reduction:** Both mindfulness and meditation are known for their stress-reducing properties. They can help ease the emotional burden of a cancer diagnosis and treatment.

2. **Emotional Balance:** These practices can promote emotional balance, allowing you to navigate the ups and downs of your cancer journey with greater equanimity.

3. **Improved Focus:** Mindfulness and meditation can enhance your ability to concentrate and make clear decisions, even in the face of uncertainty.

4. **Pain Management:** Some individuals find that mindfulness and meditation help them manage cancer-related pain and discomfort.

Incorporating Mindfulness and Meditation

Incorporating mindfulness and meditation into your daily life can be a deeply rewarding and transformative experience:

1. **Start Small:** Begin with short sessions, just a few minutes a day, and gradually increase the duration as you become more comfortable with the practice.
2. **Guided Sessions:** Consider using guided meditation apps or recordings to help you get started. These provide structure and instruction for your practice.
3. **Quiet Space:** Find a quiet, comfortable space where you can sit or lie down without distractions. Create an environment conducive to relaxation.
4. **Body Awareness:** Pay attention to your body, its sensations, and your breath. Breath awareness is a fundamental aspect of mindfulness and meditation.
5. **Thought Observation:** Observe your thoughts without judgment. When your mind wanders, gently bring your focus back to your breath or a chosen point of focus.
6. **Consistency:** Consistency is key. Make mindfulness and meditation a daily habit to reap the full benefits of these practices.

Mindfulness in Daily Life

Mindfulness isn't limited to formal meditation sessions; it can be infused into your daily activities:

1. **Eating Mindfully:** Pay attention to the flavors, textures, and sensations of each bite during meals. This can enhance your enjoyment of food and promote healthy eating habits.
2. **Walking Mindfully:** When you walk, be fully present in the experience. Feel the ground beneath your feet, the air against your skin, and the rhythm of your steps.
3. **Breathing Mindfully:** Take moments throughout the day to focus on your breath. Deep, mindful breaths can instantly calm your nervous system.

Benefits for Your Cancer Journey

Mindfulness and meditation can offer specific benefits as you navigate your cancer journey:

1. **Emotional Support:** These practices can provide emotional support, helping you manage fear, anxiety, and depression.
2. **Pain Management:** Mindfulness techniques, such as breath awareness and visualization, can be effective tools for managing pain.
3. **Communication:** Enhanced mindfulness can improve communication with your healthcare team, helping you express your needs and concerns more effectively.
4. **Resilience:** Cultivating mindfulness and meditation can boost your resilience and help you face the

challenges of cancer with greater strength and inner peace.

A Journey of Self-Discovery

Your journey with mindfulness and meditation is a personal one:

1. **Self-Exploration:** As you engage in these practices, you may discover new insights about yourself, your thoughts, and your emotions.
2. **Adaptation:** Tailor your mindfulness and meditation practice to your needs. What works for one person may not work for another, so adapt your approach accordingly.
3. **Patience:** Be patient with yourself as you embark on this journey. The benefits of mindfulness and meditation may become more apparent over time.

Mindfulness as a Companion

Think of mindfulness and meditation as companions on your cancer journey, offering solace, resilience, and moments of profound peace. Whether you seek refuge from stress, a means to manage symptoms, or simply a way to find stillness within, these practices can be a source of comfort and strength.

CHAPTER SIX
MAINTAINING PHYSICAL HEALTH

6.1 Exercise and Cancer

The idea of engaging in exercise while battling cancer may seem counterintuitive, but the benefits of physical activity are increasingly recognized as an essential component of cancer care. In this section, we'll explore how exercise can play a vital role in your cancer journey, contributing to your overall well-being and quality of life.

The Benefits of Exercise

Exercise offers a multitude of benefits that can positively impact your physical and emotional health during your cancer journey:

1. **Strength and Endurance:** Regular exercise can enhance muscle strength and improve overall endurance, helping you better tolerate cancer treatments.
2. **Energy Levels:** Physical activity can boost your energy levels, counteracting the fatigue that often accompanies cancer and its treatments.
3. **Mood Enhancement:** Exercise triggers the release of endorphins, your body's natural mood elevators, which can reduce stress, anxiety, and depression.

4. **Pain Management:** Some individuals find that exercise helps with pain management, particularly in cases of musculoskeletal discomfort.

5. **Immune Function:** Regular physical activity may support a healthier immune system, aiding your body's ability to cope with infections and treatment side effects.

6. **Improved Sleep:** Exercise can contribute to better sleep patterns, leading to enhanced overall well-being.

Consult Your Healthcare Team

Before embarking on an exercise program, it's essential to consult with your healthcare team, including your oncologist and a physical therapist. They can help you determine a safe and suitable exercise plan tailored to your specific needs and treatment.

Types of Exercise

The ideal exercise program for you may vary depending on your cancer type, treatment phase, and individual preferences. Consider the following options:

1. **Aerobic Exercise:** Activities like walking, swimming, cycling, and dancing can improve cardiovascular health and overall endurance.
2. **Strength Training:** Resistance exercises, using body weight, resistance bands, or free weights, can help build muscle and maintain strength.
3. **Flexibility and Balance:** Yoga, Tai Chi, and stretching exercises can enhance flexibility, balance, and reduce muscle tension.
4. **Mind-Body Practices:** Mindfulness-based exercises like yoga and Tai Chi offer the dual benefits of physical activity and relaxation.

Starting Slow and Staying Consistent

When incorporating exercise into your daily routine, remember to start slowly and progress at your own pace. Here are some tips:

1. **Set Realistic Goals:** Begin with achievable goals and gradually increase the intensity and duration of your workouts as your fitness level improves.
2. **Listen to Your Body:** Pay close attention to how your body responds to exercise. If you experience pain,

dizziness, or other discomfort, consult your healthcare team.

3. **Variety:** Incorporate a variety of exercises to keep things interesting and target different muscle groups.
4. **Consistency:** Aim for regular, consistent exercise. Even short sessions a few times a week can yield benefits.

Emotional Well-Being

Exercise not only impacts your physical health but also contributes to your emotional well-being:

1. **Mood Enhancement:** Regular physical activity can alleviate stress, anxiety, and depression, providing emotional support during your cancer journey.
2. **Social Connection:** Consider engaging in group exercise classes or activities with friends and family. The social aspect can be uplifting.

Celebrate Progress

Every step you take on your exercise journey is a celebration of your strength and determination:

1. **Milestones:** Celebrate milestones, no matter how small. Each achievement is a testament to your resilience.

2. **Positive Reinforcement:** Focus on the positive changes you experience in your body and mind as you incorporate exercise into your life.
3. **Self-Compassion:** Be kind to yourself if you miss a workout or face challenges. Your journey is unique, and setbacks are a natural part of the process.

A Journey of Empowerment

Engaging in exercise during your cancer journey is a powerful way to take an active role in your well-being:

1. **Empowerment:** By participating in regular physical activity, you're demonstrating your determination to live your life to the fullest.
2. **Control:** Exercise gives you a sense of control over your body and your health, even when faced with the uncertainties of cancer.
3. **Quality of Life:** Embrace the opportunity to enhance your overall quality of life and well-being.

Your Unique Journey

Your exercise journey is a personal and unique path. Whether you engage in gentle stretching, brisk walks, or more intense workouts, know that every step you take is a testament to your strength and resilience.

6.2 Sleep and Rest

Quality sleep and rest are fundamental aspects of your well-being, particularly during a challenging time like your cancer journey. In this section, we'll explore the importance of sleep, share strategies to improve your sleep quality, and emphasize the significance of rest in your overall health and recovery.

Understanding the Importance of Sleep

Quality sleep is essential for your physical, emotional, and mental health, especially during your cancer journey:

1. **Physical Healing:** Sleep supports your body's natural healing processes, including tissue repair and immune system function.
2. **Energy Restoration:** Restorative sleep replenishes your energy levels, helping you feel more awake and alert during the day.
3. **Emotional Well-Being:** A good night's sleep can improve mood, reduce stress, and enhance your ability to cope with the emotional challenges of cancer.
4. **Cognitive Function:** Sleep is crucial for cognitive functions such as memory, concentration, and decision-making.
5. **Pain Management:** Adequate sleep can help manage pain and discomfort, making it an essential component of your overall pain management strategy.

Improving Sleep Quality

If cancer treatments, symptoms, or emotional distress are affecting your sleep, there are strategies you can employ to improve your sleep quality:

1. **Sleep Hygiene:** Establish a regular sleep schedule by going to bed and waking up at the same times each day. Create a calming bedtime routine to signal your body that it's time to wind down.

2. **Comfortable Sleep Environment:** Ensure your sleep space is comfortable and conducive to rest. Invest in a good mattress and pillows and control the room temperature and lighting to suit your preferences.

3. **Limit Stimulants:** Reduce caffeine and alcohol intake, particularly in the hours leading up to bedtime, as these substances can interfere with sleep.

4. **Mindfulness and Relaxation:** Practice relaxation techniques such as deep breathing, meditation, or progressive muscle relaxation to calm your mind and body before sleep.

5. **Limit Screen Time:** Avoid screens (phones, tablets, computers, and TVs) at least an hour before bedtime, as the blue light emitted can disrupt your sleep-wake cycle.

6. **Address Anxiety and Stress:** Seek support from a therapist, counselor, or support group to manage anxiety and stress that may be interfering with your sleep.

The Value of Rest

While sleep is crucial, rest extends beyond nighttime slumber. Rest during the day is equally important:

1. **Short Naps:** Short, daytime naps can be refreshing and provide an energy boost. Aim for naps of 20-30 minutes to avoid grogginess.
2. **Pacing Yourself:** Manage your energy levels by pacing yourself throughout the day. Listen to your body and rest when needed.
3. **Emotional Rest:** Recognize the importance of emotional rest. Take breaks from stressful situations and engage in activities that bring you joy and relaxation.
4. **Prioritize Self-Care:** Self-care practices, such as gentle activities, hobbies, or spending time with loved ones, contribute to emotional and mental rest.

Seeking Professional Help

If sleep disturbances persist and significantly impact your quality of life, consult your healthcare team. They can provide guidance, assess underlying causes, and offer solutions to improve your sleep and rest.

Your Journey to Healing

Remember that your sleep and rest are vital components of your healing journey:

1. **Self-Compassion:** Be gentle with yourself if sleep disruptions occur. Understand that it's normal to have occasional sleep challenges, especially during times of stress.
2. **Quality Over Quantity:** Focus on the quality of your sleep and rest rather than the quantity. Restorative sleep and well-timed breaks can be more beneficial than prolonged, restless nights.
3. **Advocacy:** Advocate for your sleep needs and communicate with your healthcare team about any issues you may be facing.

A Path to Well-Being

Quality sleep and rest are not luxuries but essential components of your overall well-being. By prioritizing your sleep and embracing moments of rest, you empower your body and mind to heal and thrive during your cancer journey.

6.3 Immune System Support

Your immune system plays a vital role in your overall health, especially during your cancer journey. In this section, we'll explore strategies to support and strengthen your immune system, helping you better cope with treatments and enhance your overall well-being.

Understanding the Immune System

Your immune system is a complex network of cells, tissues, and organs that defends your body against infections, illnesses, and even cancer. Cancer and its treatments can put stress on your immune system, making it crucial to support and fortify its function.

Diet and Nutrition

A well-balanced diet is essential for immune system support:

1. **Fruits and Vegetables:** These are rich in antioxidants, vitamins, and minerals that can boost your immune system. Aim for a colorful variety to ensure a wide range of nutrients.
2. **Protein:** Lean proteins like poultry, fish, tofu, and legumes provide amino acids necessary for immune function.
3. **Whole Grains:** Choose whole grains like brown rice, quinoa, and whole wheat for a steady supply of energy and nutrients.

4. **Healthy Fats:** Incorporate sources of healthy fats, such as avocados, nuts, seeds, and olive oil, which have anti-inflammatory properties.
5. **Hydration:** Staying well-hydrated is crucial for overall health. Water supports bodily functions, including immune system function.

Supplements and Herbs

While a well-rounded diet should provide most of the nutrients you need, supplements and herbs may be beneficial in some cases:

1. **Vitamin D:** Adequate vitamin D levels are important for immune function. Your healthcare team can assess your levels and recommend supplements if necessary.
2. **Probiotics:** These beneficial bacteria can support gut health, which is closely linked to immune function.
3. **Herbs:** Certain herbs, like echinacea and astragalus, are believed to have immune-boosting properties. Consult with your healthcare team before using herbal supplements.

Hygiene and Infection Prevention

Maintaining good hygiene practices can help prevent infections, which can be particularly important during cancer treatment when your immune system may be compromised:

1. **Handwashing:** Wash your hands regularly with soap and water, especially before eating and after using the restroom.
2. **Avoid Sick Individuals:** Limit exposure to individuals who are sick and ask loved ones to practice good hygiene if they're ill.
3. **Vaccinations:** Stay up to date with recommended vaccinations to protect against preventable diseases.

Physical Activity

Regular exercise can contribute to a healthy immune system:

1. **Moderate Activity:** Engage in moderate-intensity exercises like walking, swimming, or cycling to promote immune function and overall health.
2. **Avoid Overexertion:** Listen to your body and avoid overexertion, which can weaken your immune system.
3. **Consult Your Healthcare Team:** Always consult your healthcare team before starting or modifying an exercise routine, especially during active treatment.

Stress Management

Chronic stress can weaken your immune system. Here are some strategies to manage stress:

1. **Mindfulness and Relaxation:** Practice mindfulness meditation, deep breathing exercises, or progressive muscle relaxation to reduce stress.
2. **Counseling and Support:** Seek emotional support from a therapist, counselor, or support group to help manage stress and anxiety.
3. **Hobbies and Interests:** Engage in activities you enjoy relieving stress and promote well-being.

Quality Sleep

Adequate sleep is crucial for immune system support:

1. **Sleep Hygiene:** Create a sleep-conducive environment by keeping your bedroom dark, quiet, and comfortable.
2. **Routine:** Establish a regular sleep schedule and avoid stimulating activities before bedtime.
3. **Restorative Sleep:** Prioritize quality rest to allow your body to repair and rejuvenate.

Consult Your Healthcare Team

Before making significant changes to your diet, exercise routine, or supplement regimen, it's essential to consult with your healthcare team. They can provide personalized guidance based on your specific treatment and medical history.

A Holistic Approach to Well-Being

Supporting your immune system is an integral part of your overall well-being during your cancer journey:

1. **Personalized Approach:** Work with your healthcare team to develop a personalized plan for immune system support that suits your specific needs.

2. **Patience:** Understand that strengthening your immune system takes time. Be patient with yourself and your body's healing process.

3. **Empowerment:** By taking an active role in supporting your immune system, you empower yourself on your journey to healing.

Your immune system is a powerful ally in your fight against cancer. By nurturing and supporting it through these strategies, you can enhance your overall health and well-being during this challenging time.

6.4 Sexual Health

Sexual health is an important aspect of your overall well-being, and it can be impacted by a cancer diagnosis and treatment. In this section, we'll discuss the challenges that may arise and offer guidance on maintaining a healthy and fulfilling sexual life during your cancer journey.

Understanding the Impact of Cancer on Sexual Health

Cancer and its treatments can affect various aspects of sexual health:

1. **Physical Changes:** Surgery, radiation, chemotherapy, and hormone therapy can lead to physical changes that may impact sexual function, such as vaginal dryness, erectile dysfunction, or changes in libido.
2. **Emotional Impact:** The emotional toll of cancer, including fear, anxiety, and depression, can affect your sexual desire and intimacy.
3. **Body Image:** Changes in body image due to surgery or treatment side effects may lead to self-consciousness and impact your self-esteem in intimate situations.
4. **Communication:** Open and honest communication about your feelings and concerns regarding sexual health is essential, both with your partner and your healthcare team.

Talking to Your Healthcare Team

Your healthcare team can provide guidance and solutions to address sexual health concerns:

1. **Raise Concerns:** Don't hesitate to bring up any sexual health concerns with your oncologist or nurse. They are trained to discuss and offer solutions for these issues.

2. **Ask Questions:** If you have questions about the impact of treatments on your sexual health, seek clarification from your healthcare provider.

3. **Explore Options:** Discuss potential treatments or strategies that can help mitigate the sexual side effects of cancer treatments.

Counseling and Support

Seeking emotional support and counseling can be invaluable in addressing the emotional and relational aspects of sexual health:

1. **Therapist or Counselor:** Consider working with a therapist or counselor experienced in sexual health or oncology. They can help you navigate the emotional challenges you may be facing.
2. **Support Groups:** Joining a cancer support group can provide a safe space to discuss your concerns and connect with others facing similar challenges.

Intimacy and Communication

Maintaining intimacy and open communication with your partner is essential:

1. **Communication:** Talk openly with your partner about your feelings, desires, and concerns. Honest communication can strengthen your connection.
2. **Empathy:** Understand that your partner may also be experiencing their own emotional responses to your cancer journey. Show empathy and support for each other.
3. **Intimacy Beyond Sex:** Remember that intimacy is not solely about sexual activity. Emotional intimacy, affection, and closeness are equally important components of a fulfilling relationship.

Exploring Solutions

There are various solutions and strategies to address sexual health challenges:

1. **Medical Solutions:** Consult with your healthcare provider about medical options such as medications, hormone replacement therapy, or devices that may help address sexual issues.
2. **Sexual Therapy:** A qualified sex therapist can provide guidance and exercises to improve sexual function and intimacy.
3. **Lubricants and Moisturizers:** Products designed to alleviate vaginal dryness can enhance comfort and pleasure during intimacy.
4. **Adaptation:** Explore different sexual positions or techniques that may be more comfortable and enjoyable.
o **Patience:** Understand that it may take time to find solutions that work for you. Be patient with yourself and your partner as you navigate these challenges together.

Self-Care and Self-Compassion

Above all, practice self-care and self-compassion as you address sexual health challenges:

1. **Self-Acceptance:** Embrace your body and its changes with self-acceptance and self-love.

2. **Empowerment:** Recognize that you could adapt and find ways to enjoy a fulfilling sexual life.

3. **Seeking Pleasure:** Focus on pleasure and connection rather than perfection. Rediscover the joy of physical intimacy without putting undue pressure on yourself.

Your Unique Journey

Your sexual health journey is unique, and it may involve challenges and adaptations. By addressing these issues with openness, empathy, and support, you can maintain a fulfilling and satisfying sexual life during your cancer journey.

CHAPTER SEVEN
PRACTICAL TIPS FOR DAILY LIVING

7.1 Organizing Medical Records

Amid the complexities of a cancer diagnosis and treatment, organizing your medical records is a practical step that can streamline your healthcare journey, improve communication with your healthcare team, and empower you to make informed decisions. In this section, we'll explore tips and strategies to help you efficiently manage your medical records.

Why Organizing Medical Records Matters

Medical records are a crucial part of your cancer care:

1. **Comprehensive Understanding:** Well-organized records provide a comprehensive view of your medical history, treatments, and outcomes.
2. **Effective Communication:** Clear and organized records facilitate communication with your healthcare team, ensuring they have accurate information for your care.
3. **Empowerment:** Access to your medical records empowers you to actively participate in your care decisions, ask informed questions, and advocate for your needs.

Creating a Medical Record System

Establishing an organized medical record system can simplify the management of your healthcare information:

1. **Designate a Binder or Digital Folder:** Choose a physical binder or create a digital folder dedicated to your medical records.
2. **Sections:** Organize your records into sections for different types of information, such as diagnosis, treatment plans, lab results, and correspondence.
3. **Chronological Order:** Arrange documents within each section in chronological order, starting with the most recent.
4. **Labels and Dividers:** Use labels and dividers to easily locate specific documents or sections within your record.

Documenting Information

Accurate and comprehensive documentation is key:

1. **Copies of Reports:** Include copies of medical reports, test results, pathology reports, and imaging studies in your record.
2. Treatment Plans: Keep records of treatment plans, including medications, dosages, and schedules.
3. **Doctor's Notes:** Include notes from your healthcare appointments, summarizing discussions, treatment recommendations, and follow-up plans.
4. **Correspondence:** Save copies of emails or letters related to your medical care, including communication with your healthcare team, insurance providers, or billing inquiries.

Digital Record Keeping

Digital record keeping can be efficient and easily accessible:

1. **Secure Storage:** Use secure digital platforms, such as cloud storage services or password-protected files, to store electronic copies of your records.
2. **Backup:** Regularly back up your digital records to prevent data loss.
3. **Scanning:** Scan physical documents to create digital copies for easy access and sharing with healthcare providers.

4. **Password Protection:** Ensure that digital records are protected with strong, unique passwords.

Taking Notes

During medical appointments, take notes to document important information:

1. **Questions:** List questions you want to ask your healthcare provider.
2. **Answers:** Record the answers and recommendations provided by your healthcare team.
3. **Clarifications:** If something is unclear, ask for clarification or have your provider explain in simpler terms.

Maintaining an Appointment Calendar

Keep a calendar to track appointments and follow-up dates:

1. **Appointment Details:** Include the date, time, location, and purpose of each appointment.
2. **Reminders:** Set reminders for upcoming appointments to ensure you don't miss them.

Sharing Information

Share your organized medical records as needed:

Healthcare Team: Provide copies of your records to your primary care physician and specialists involved in your care.

Emergency Contacts: Share a summary of your records with emergency contacts or family members who may need access in case of an emergency.

Privacy and Security

Protect your medical records to maintain privacy and security:

1. **Access Control:** Limit access to your records to trusted individuals and healthcare providers.
2. **Password Protection:** Secure digital records with strong, unique passwords.

3. **Secure Storage:** Store physical records in a safe and secure location.

Regular Updates

Keep your medical records up to date:

1. **Routine Updates:** Add new information as you receive it, such as test results or treatment changes.
2. **Review:** Periodically review your records to ensure accuracy and completeness.

Empowering Your Healthcare Journey

Organizing your medical records empowers you to actively participate in your healthcare journey, communicate effectively with your healthcare team, and make informed decisions. By implementing these strategies, you'll have a comprehensive and accessible record of your cancer care, supporting a smoother and more informed healthcare experience.

7.2 Managing Medications

Medications are a crucial component of cancer treatment and symptom management. Properly managing your medications ensures their effectiveness, minimizes side effects, and contributes to your overall well-being. In this section, we'll explore strategies for organizing and safely managing your medications during your cancer journey.

Understanding Your Medications

Knowledge is power when it comes to your medications:

1. **Know Your Medications:** Familiarize yourself with the names, purposes, dosages, and potential side effects of each medication you're prescribed.
2. **Create a Medication List:** Maintain a list of your medications, both prescription and over the counter, and keep it up to date.
3. **Ask Questions:** Don't hesitate to ask your healthcare team questions about your medications, including how they work and what to expect.

Organization and Storage

Efficient organization and proper storage are essential for medication management:

1. **Designate a Medication Space:** Set up a specific area, such as a medicine cabinet or a dedicated drawer, for your medications.

2. **Separate Medications:** Keep medications in separate containers or drawers to prevent mix-ups.

3. **Check Expiration Dates:** Regularly check the expiration dates on your medications and dispose of any that have expired.

4. **Temperature Control:** Store medications according to their recommended temperature requirements. Some may need refrigeration, while others should be kept at room temperature.

Medication Schedule

Adhering to a consistent medication schedule is critical:

1. **Set Alarms or Reminders:** Use alarms on your phone or medication reminder apps to ensure you take your medications on time.
2. **Use a Pill Organizer:** Pill organizers with compartments for each day and time can help you keep track of your medications.
3. **Follow Instructions:** Take medications exactly as prescribed by your healthcare provider. Don't skip doses or alter dosages without consulting them.
4. **Record Taking Medications:** Consider keeping a daily medication journal to track when you take each medication and note any side effects.

Medication Interactions

Be aware of potential interactions between medications:

1. **Inform Your Healthcare Team:** Always inform your healthcare team about all medications you're taking, including vitamins, supplements, and over-the-counter drugs.
2. **Ask About Interactions:** If you're prescribed a new medication, ask your healthcare provider about potential interactions with your existing medications.

3. **Pharmacist Consultation:** Consult with your pharmacist for insights into potential interactions and guidance on safe medication use.

Side Effects and Adverse Reactions

Understanding and managing medication side effects is crucial:

1. **Side Effect Awareness:** Be aware of common side effects associated with your medications. Report any unusual or severe side effects to your healthcare team.
2. **Addressing Side Effects:** Discuss side effect management strategies with your healthcare provider. They may adjust your medication or recommend supportive care.

Medication Disposal

Properly disposing of medications is important for safety:

1. **Follow Disposal Guidelines:** Dispose of expired or unused medications following recommended guidelines from your healthcare provider or local pharmacy.
2. **Medication Take-Back Programs:** Many communities offer medication take-back programs or events to safely dispose of medications.

Advocacy and Communication

Effective communication with your healthcare team is key to medication management:

Be Your Own Advocate: Take an active role in your healthcare by asking questions, expressing concerns, and advocating for your needs.

Clear Communication: Inform your healthcare provider of any changes in your health, new symptoms, or difficulties with your medications promptly.

Second Opinions: If you have doubts or concerns about your treatment plan or medication regimen, consider seeking a second opinion.

A Comprehensive Approach to Care

Managing medications is an integral part of your cancer care journey:

1. **Empowerment:** By understanding your medications and actively participating in their management, you empower yourself in your healthcare decisions.
2. **Quality of Life:** Effective medication management can enhance your quality of life by controlling symptoms and supporting treatment effectiveness.
3. **Communication:** Open and transparent communication with your healthcare team ensures you receive the best care possible.

Your dedication to properly managing your medications is a testament to your commitment to your health and well-being during your cancer journey.

7.3 Financial and Insurance Guidance

Coping with cancer is not just a physical and emotional challenge; it can also present financial and insurance-related concerns. In this section, we'll explore strategies to help you navigate the complex landscape of medical expenses, insurance coverage, and financial planning during your cancer journey.

Understanding Your Insurance

A clear understanding of your insurance coverage is essential:

1. **Policy Review:** Thoroughly review your insurance policy, including its coverage, limitations, deductibles, and co-pays. Familiarize yourself with your plan's terms and conditions.
2. **Contact Your Provider:** If you have questions or need clarification, contact your insurance provider or a patient advocate for assistance.
3. **Network Providers:** Utilize in-network healthcare providers whenever possible to minimize out-of-pocket expenses.
4. **Prior Authorization:** Understand when and how to obtain prior authorization for treatments and medications to ensure coverage.

Financial Planning

Developing a financial plan can provide stability during a challenging time:

1. **Budget:** Create a budget that outlines your income, expenses, and savings. Adjust your budget to accommodate medical expenses.

2. **Emergency Fund:** If possible, establish an emergency fund to cover unexpected costs related to your cancer care.

3. **Financial Advisor:** Consider consulting a financial advisor who specializes in healthcare planning for personalized guidance.

Financial Assistance Programs

Explore financial assistance programs that may be available to you:

1. **Charities and Foundations:** Many organizations offer financial assistance for cancer patients, including help with medical bills, transportation, and lodging.
2. **Government Programs:** Investigate government programs such as Medicaid or Supplemental Security Income (SSI) if you meet eligibility criteria.
3. **Clinical Trials:** Some clinical trials cover the cost of experimental treatments and associated medical expenses.
4. **Hospital Programs:** Inquire about financial assistance programs offered by your treatment center or hospital.

Open Communication

Maintaining open communication about your financial concerns is essential:

1. **Discuss Costs:** Don't hesitate to discuss the financial aspects of your care with your healthcare team. They may have insights or suggestions.
2. **Negotiation:** If you're facing financial hardship, negotiate with your healthcare providers and insurers for manageable payment plans or reduced fees.

3. **Appeal Denials:** If a claim is denied, appeal the decision. Your healthcare team can assist with this process.

Prescription Assistance

Prescription medications can be costly, but assistance may be available:

1. **Patient Assistance Programs**: Some pharmaceutical companies offer patient assistance programs that provide medications at reduced or no cost to eligible individuals.
2. **Generic Options:** When possible, inquire about generic versions of prescribed medications, as they are often more affordable.
3. **Pharmacy Discounts:** Explore pharmacy discount programs or apps that may provide savings on prescription medications.

Workplace Benefits

Review your workplace benefits and resources:

1. **Health Savings Accounts (HSAs) and Flexible Spending Accounts (FSAs):** If available, consider utilizing these accounts to cover medical expenses with pre-tax dollars.
2. **Employee Assistance Programs (EAPs):** EAPs may offer financial counseling and resources to help you cope with financial challenges.
3. **Short-Term Disability:** Investigate short-term disability benefits if you need to take time off work during your treatment.

Legal and Financial Documentation

Ensure that your legal and financial documents are up to date:

1. **Advance Directives:** Create or update advance directives to specify your healthcare wishes in case you're unable to make decisions.
2. **Power of Attorney:** Designate a trusted individual to handle financial matters on your behalf if necessary.
3. **Wills and Estate Planning:** Review your will and estate plan and make any necessary updates.

Advocacy and Support

Consider seeking help from a financial counselor or patient advocate:

1. **Patient Advocates:** Many hospitals have patient advocates who can help you navigate insurance and financial matters.
2. **Cancer Support Organizations:** Connect with cancer support organizations and local resources that offer financial guidance and support.

Your Well-Being Matters

Remember that managing your financial and insurance concerns is part of your holistic well-being:

1. **Stress Management:** Managing financial stress is essential for your overall health. Utilize stress-reduction techniques such as meditation, mindfulness, or counseling.
2. **Support Network:** Lean on your support network, including friends and family, for emotional and practical assistance during this challenging time.
3. **Self-Advocacy:** Be a proactive advocate for yourself. Don't hesitate to seek help and guidance when needed.

Navigating the financial and insurance aspects of cancer care can be challenging, but with careful planning and advocacy, you can ease the burden on yourself and your loved ones.

7.4 Legal and Estate Planning

Facing a cancer diagnosis is a challenging journey that may prompt you to consider important legal and estate planning matters. In this section, we'll discuss the crucial steps you can take to ensure your wishes are respected, your loved ones are provided for, and your affairs are in order during your cancer journey.

Advance Directives

Advance directives are legal documents that outline your healthcare preferences in case you become unable to make decisions. These documents include:

1. **Living Will:** A living will specify your preferences for medical treatments, such as resuscitation or life support, in case you can't communicate your wishes.
2. **Healthcare Power of Attorney:** Designate a trusted person as your healthcare proxy to make medical decisions on your behalf if you can't.
3. **Do-Not-Resuscitate (DNR) Order:** Specify whether you want cardiopulmonary resuscitation (CPR) or not in case your heart or breathing stops.
4. **POLST (Physician Orders for Life-Sustaining Treatment):** A POLST form provides specific medical orders and complements your advance directives. It's particularly useful for individuals with serious illnesses.

Legal Counsel

Consult an attorney experienced in estate planning and healthcare law to help you create and validate these important documents. They can also assist with:

1. **Wills:** A will outline how your assets should be distributed after your passing. It can also specify guardianship arrangements if you have minor children.
2. **Trusts:** Consider setting up trusts to manage and distribute assets according to your wishes, potentially avoiding probate.
3. **Financial Power of Attorney:** Designate someone to manage your financial affairs if you're unable to do so.

Regular Updates

Review and update your legal documents periodically, especially after major life events like a cancer diagnosis, treatment changes, or significant financial changes.

Communication

Discuss your end-of-life preferences and legal documents with your loved ones:

1. **Family Discussions:** Engage in open conversations with your family about your wishes and the role each person will play in carrying them out.
2. **Access to Documents: Ensure** that your healthcare proxy and loved ones know where to find your legal documents when needed.

Beneficiary Designations

Review and update beneficiary designations on insurance policies, retirement accounts, and other financial assets to ensure they align with your current wishes.

Consider Financial Planning

Estate planning may involve financial considerations:

1. **Life Insurance:** Evaluate whether life insurance is necessary to provide for your loved ones or cover financial obligations.

2. **Long-Term Care Insurance:** Explore long-term care insurance options, as cancer treatment may lead to long-term care needs.

Digital Estate Planning

Consider your digital assets:

1. **Digital Accounts:** Keep a record of online accounts, including usernames and passwords, in a secure place.
2. **Digital Assets:** Specify your wishes for digital assets, such as social media accounts, websites, and online subscriptions, in your estate planning documents.

End-of-Life Decisions

Consider your preferences regarding end-of-life care:

1. **Hospice Care:** Explore hospice care options if they align with your end-of-life wishes.
2. **Palliative Care:** Palliative care focuses on improving quality of life for individuals with serious illnesses. Discuss whether it's appropriate for you.

Document Storage

Store your legal and estate planning documents in a safe, accessible location:

1. **Secure Location:** Keep physical copies in a secure location, such as a home safe or bank safe deposit box.
2. **Digital Copies:** Create digital copies and store them in a secure, password-protected digital vault or share them with a trusted person.

Legal and Emotional Support

Engage with an attorney who can guide you through the legal aspects of planning and consult with mental health professionals or support groups to help you cope with the emotional aspects.

Your Legacy

Planning your legal and estate affairs is an act of love and responsibility. It ensures that your wishes are honored, your loved ones are supported, and your legacy endures.

CHAPTER EIGHT
SUPPORT FOR CAREGIVERS

8.1 The Role of Caregivers

Caring for someone with cancer is a profound act of love and support, but it can also be emotionally and physically demanding. In this section, we'll explore the crucial role caregivers play in a cancer patient's journey and provide guidance on how to navigate the challenges and responsibilities that come with it.

The Caregiver's Role

As a caregiver, your role is multifaceted and essential:

1. **Emotional Support:** Provide emotional support and a reassuring presence to the person with cancer. Listen, offer comfort, and be empathetic to their feelings and concerns.

2. **Practical Assistance:** Assist with daily tasks such as cooking, cleaning, transportation to medical appointments, and medication management.

3. **Advocacy:** Act as an advocate for the person with cancer, ensuring their voice is heard and their needs are met within the healthcare system.

4. **Communication:** Help facilitate clear and open communication between the patient and their healthcare team. Take notes during medical

appointments and ask questions on behalf of the patient when necessary.

5. **Personal Care:** Assist with personal care needs, such as bathing, dressing, and mobility support, if required.

6. **Medication Management:** Help manage medications, including ensuring they are taken as prescribed and refilled on time.

7. **Nutritional Support:** Assist with meal planning and preparation to ensure the patient is receiving adequate nutrition during treatment.

8. **Emotional Well-Being:** Encourage activities that promote emotional well-being, such as engaging in hobbies, spending time with loved ones, and seeking counseling or support groups.

Self-Care for Caregivers

Caring for someone with cancer can be emotionally and physically taxing. It's vital for caregivers to prioritize self-care:

1. **Accept Help:** Don't hesitate to accept help from friends, family, or support organizations. You don't have to do everything on your own.
2. **Respite:** Take regular breaks to rest and recharge. Caregiver burnout can negatively impact both you and the person you're caring for.
3. **Support Groups:** Consider joining a caregiver support group to connect with others who understand your challenges.
4. **Set Boundaries:** Establish boundaries to protect your physical and emotional well-being. Communicate your needs to others.
5. **Professional Help:** Seek professional counseling or therapy if you're feeling overwhelmed or experiencing caregiver stress.

Communication and Empathy

Effective communication is key to providing the best care and support:

1. **Listen Actively:** Listen attentively to the patient's concerns and feelings. Sometimes, they may simply need someone to talk to.

2. **Empathy:** Put yourself in their shoes and try to understand their perspective and emotions. Empathy fosters a deeper connection.
3. **Ask for Input:** Involve the person with cancer in decision-making about their care whenever possible. Respect their autonomy and preferences.

Supporting the Caregiver-Patient Relationship

Maintaining a strong caregiver-patient relationship is crucial:

1. **Open Dialogue:** Foster open and honest communication with the person you're caring for. Encourage them to express their needs and concerns.
2. **Patience:** Understand that both you and the patient may experience moments of frustration or stress. Patience and understanding are key.
3. **Quality Time:** Spend quality time together outside of the caregiving context. Enjoy activities that bring joy and relaxation.

Advocacy

As a caregiver, you may find yourself advocating for the patient:

1. **Learn About the Illness:** Educate yourself about the person's specific cancer type and treatment plan. Knowledge empowers effective advocacy.

2. **Ask Questions:** Don't hesitate to ask the healthcare team questions, seek clarification, and advocate for the patient's needs and preferences.
3. **Document Care:** Keep records of medical appointments, test results, and treatment plans. This documentation can be valuable for continuity of care.

A Supportive Network

Lean on your support network:

1. **Friends and Family:** Share your feelings and concerns with trusted friends and family members. They can provide emotional support.
2. **Support Organizations:** Connect with cancer caregiver support organizations or local resources that offer guidance and assistance.

Celebrating Small Victories

Celebrate the small victories along the way:

1. **Milestones:** Acknowledge treatment milestones, positive moments, and personal achievements in the cancer journey.
2. **Resilience:** Recognize your resilience as a caregiver and the strength you bring to the person's life.

Your Role Matters

As a caregiver, you play a vital role in the cancer journey. Your love, support, and dedication make a profound difference in the life of the person you're caring for. Remember to care for yourself, seek help when needed, and embrace the privilege of making a positive impact on someone's life during a challenging time.

8.2 Self-Care for Caregivers

Caring for a loved one with cancer is a noble and compassionate act, but it can also be emotionally and physically draining. It's essential to remember that taking care of yourself is not selfish; it's necessary for providing the best care to your loved one. In this section, we'll explore strategies for self-care that can help you maintain your well-being while supporting your loved one through their cancer journey.

The Importance of Self-Care

Self-care is not a luxury; it's a fundamental aspect of your role as a caregiver:

1. **Resilience:** Prioritizing self-care enhances your emotional and physical resilience, allowing you to better handle the challenges of caregiving.
2. **Effective Support:** By taking care of yourself, you're better equipped to provide effective and compassionate care to your loved one.
3. **Role Model:** Demonstrating self-care sets a positive example for your loved one and encourages them to prioritize their own well-being.

Self-Care Strategies

Accept Help: Don't hesitate to accept assistance from friends, family, or support organizations. Let others share the caregiving responsibilities to lighten your load.

1. **Set Boundaries:** Establish clear boundaries to protect your physical and emotional well-being. Communicate your limits to others and respect them.

2. **Respite:** Take regular breaks to rest and recharge. Caregiver burnout can harm both you and your loved one. Use these breaks for activities you enjoy or simply to relax.

3. **Support Groups:** Join a caregiver support group to connect with others who understand your challenges. Sharing experiences and tips can be immensely comforting.

4. **Professional Help:** Seek professional counseling or therapy if you're feeling overwhelmed, stressed, or anxious. A therapist can provide coping strategies and emotional support.

5. **Physical Activity:** Engage in regular physical activity, even if it's just a short walk. Exercise can boost your mood, reduce stress, and improve your overall well-being.

6. **Healthy Eating:** Maintain a balanced diet to ensure you have the energy and nutrition you need. Avoid excessive caffeine or alcohol, as they can contribute to stress and sleep problems.

7. **Quality Sleep:** Prioritize quality sleep by establishing a regular sleep schedule and creating a comfortable sleep environment. Lack of sleep can affect your ability to provide care effectively.

8. **Mindfulness and Relaxation:** Practice mindfulness meditation, deep breathing exercises, or progressive muscle relaxation to manage stress and stay grounded.

9. **Hobbies and Interests:** Dedicate time to activities you enjoy and that bring you joy. It's essential to nurture your interests outside of caregiving.

10. **Delegate Tasks:** Share caregiving responsibilities with other family members or friends. Don't hesitate to delegate tasks like grocery shopping, meal preparation, or transportation.

11. **Maintain Social Connections:** Stay connected with friends and family who offer emotional support. Isolation can exacerbate caregiver stress.

12. **Celebrate Achievements:** Acknowledge your caregiving achievements and milestones. Celebrate both small and significant victories along the way.

13. **Set Realistic Expectations:** Understand that you can't control every aspect of your loved one's cancer journey. Setting realistic expectations for yourself and their progress is vital.

14. **Professional Assistance:** Consider hiring professional caregiving assistance or home healthcare services if needed. These services can provide essential relief.

Guilt and Self-Care

Many caregivers grapple with feelings of guilt when prioritizing self-care. Remember that taking care of yourself doesn't diminish your dedication or love for your loved one. It enhances your ability to provide effective and compassionate care.

Your Well-Being Matters

As a caregiver, your well-being is of utmost importance. By practicing self-care, you not only maintain your own health and resilience but also provide the best possible support to your loved one. Caregiving is a challenging journey, but with self-care, it becomes a sustainable and meaningful role in your loved one's cancer journey.

8.3 Communicating with the Patient

Effective communication is the foundation of providing meaningful support to someone living with cancer. It can foster trust, emotional well-being, and collaboration in their cancer journey. In this section, we'll explore strategies for communicating with the patient in ways that are empathetic, supportive, and respectful of their needs.

The Power of Communication

Open and empathetic communication can have a profound impact on the patient's experience:

1. **Trust:** Effective communication builds trust between you and the patient, allowing for more open and honest discussions.
2. **Emotional Support:** Listening and expressing empathy provide emotional support during a challenging time.
3. **Collaboration:** Good communication facilitates collaboration between the patient and their healthcare team, leading to better care decisions.

Active Listening

Active listening is a fundamental communication skill:

1. **Be Present:** When the patient is speaking, be fully present and attentive. Put away distractions and focus on them.

2. **Eye Contact:** Maintain eye contact to convey your interest and attention.

3. **Empathize:** Acknowledge the patient's feelings and emotions. Validate their experiences by saying things like, "I can imagine that must be difficult."

4. **Ask Open-Ended Questions:** Encourage the patient to share by asking open-ended questions that require more than a simple "yes" or "no" response.

Respect Their Preferences

Every patient is unique, and their communication preferences may vary:

1. **Preferred Communication Style:** Ask the patient about their preferred communication style. Some may want to talk openly about their condition, while others may prefer to be more private.
2. **Privacy:** Respect the patient's need for privacy and confidentiality. Don't share their health information without their consent.
3. **Timing:** Consider the timing of your conversations. Some patients may prefer to discuss their condition and treatment at specific times or in certain settings.

Navigating Difficult Conversations

Cancer may involve challenging conversations:

1. **Honesty:** Be honest and transparent, but also sensitive. Provide information in a clear and compassionate manner.
2. **Prepare:** Anticipate questions the patient may have and be prepared to provide answers or resources.
3. **Silences:** Don't be afraid of silence during a conversation. Sometimes, the patient needs time to process or gather their thoughts.

4. **Emotions:** Be prepared for emotions to surface during difficult conversations. Offer comfort and support as needed.

Empower the Patient

Empower the patient to actively participate in their healthcare:

1. **Encourage Questions:** Encourage the patient to ask questions and seek clarification. Remind them that their questions and concerns are valid.
2. **Information Sharing:** Help the patient keep track of their medical information, appointments, and treatment plans. Offer to take notes during appointments.
3. **Second Opinions:** Support the patient if they express interest in seeking a second opinion. It's a valuable step in their decision-making process.
4. **Shared Decision-Making:** Facilitate shared decision-making by discussing treatment options, risks, and benefits together.

Non-Verbal Communication

Non-verbal cues are equally important:

1. **Body Language:** Your body language should convey empathy and support. Avoid crossing your arms or appearing disinterested.

2. **Touch:** Physical touch, such as holding their hand or offering a comforting hug, can convey care and support.

3. **Facial Expressions:** Your facial expressions should match the tone of your conversation. A warm smile can provide reassurance.

Checking In Regularly

Consistent communication is key:

1. **Regular Check-Ins:** Schedule regular check-ins with the patient to see how they're feeling physically and emotionally.

2. **Be Available:** Let the patient know you're available for them whenever they need to talk or have questions.

3. **Respect Their Wishes:** Respect the patient's desire for communication frequency. Some may prefer daily check-ins, while others may need more space.

Your Role as a Listener and Supporter

As a listener and supporter, your role is invaluable:

1. **Emotional Outlet:** Provide a safe space for the patient to express their feelings and fears without judgment.

2. **Problem-Solving:** Collaborate with the patient to identify solutions to challenges they may face during their cancer journey.

3. **Celebrate Victories:** Celebrate their milestones and achievements, no matter how small. It can boost their morale.

Conclusion

Effective communication with the patient is a cornerstone of caregiving and support during their cancer journey. By listening actively, respecting their preferences, and empowering them to be active participants in their healthcare decisions, you can contribute significantly to their well-being and resilience.

8.4 Seeking Additional Support

Living with cancer or supporting a loved one through their cancer journey can be emotionally and physically taxing. Seeking additional support is not a sign of weakness; it's a wise and proactive step to ensure the well-being of both the patient and the caregiver. In this section, we'll explore various sources of support that can provide comfort, guidance, and assistance during the challenging times that come with a cancer diagnosis.

The Value of Support

Additional support can provide numerous benefits:

1. **Emotional Resilience:** Support networks offer emotional reinforcement, reducing feelings of isolation and stress.
2. **Practical Assistance:** Support can come in the form of practical help with daily tasks, transportation, and caregiving responsibilities.
3. **Information and Education:** Support groups and organizations can provide valuable information and resources to help you navigate the complexities of cancer.
4. **Wellness:** Many support resources focus on promoting physical and emotional well-being, which can be especially beneficial during cancer treatment.

Types of Additional Support

Support Groups

1. **In-Person Support Groups:** Local support groups provide a safe space for patients and caregivers to share experiences and receive emotional support.
2. **Online Support Groups:** Virtual communities allow you to connect with others facing similar challenges. They're especially useful if in-person meetings are not feasible.

Counseling and Therapy

1. **Individual Counseling:** Consider individual counseling or therapy to address the unique emotional and psychological challenges you may encounter.
2. **Family Counseling:** Family therapy can help improve communication and understanding within the family unit.

Caregiver Respite:

o **Respite Care Services:** These services provide temporary relief for caregivers, allowing you to rest and recharge while a trained professional takes over caregiving duties for a short time.

Cancer Support Organizations:

- o **Local and National Organizations**: Numerous organizations specialize in cancer support, providing information, resources, and assistance tailored to your needs.

Patient Navigators:

- o **Hospital-Based Navigators:** Many hospitals have patient navigators who can guide you through the healthcare system, answer questions, and provide emotional support.

Home Healthcare Services:

- o **Skilled Professionals:** Home healthcare services can offer skilled nursing care, physical therapy, and assistance with daily activities in the comfort of your home.

Community Resources:

- o **Local Resources:** Explore community resources such as meal delivery services, transportation assistance, and support for essential needs.

Spiritual and Faith-Based Support:

o **Chaplains:** Hospitals often have chaplains who can offer spiritual guidance and support during times of illness.

Financial Counselors:

- o **Financial Planning:** Consult financial counselors or advisors who specialize in healthcare planning to help manage medical expenses and navigate insurance.

Legal and Estate Planning Professionals:

- o **Attorneys:** Seek legal professionals experienced in estate planning to assist with legal matters and ensure your affairs are in order.

Hospice Care Services:

- o **End-of-Life Support:** Hospice care provides specialized care for individuals with terminal illnesses and focuses on maximizing quality of life.

Online Resources:

- o **Websites and Forums:** Explore reputable cancer websites and forums for information, advice, and connections to others who have faced similar challenges.

Advocating for Yourself

Advocating for your needs and seeking support is a proactive step:

1. **Communicate:** Share your needs and concerns with your healthcare team. They can connect you with appropriate resources.

2. **Ask Questions:** Don't hesitate to ask questions and seek assistance. There are resources available to help you navigate your cancer journey.

3. **Research:** Research support options in your area and online. You may discover local organizations and resources that can provide valuable assistance.

Your Well-Being Matters

Remember that seeking additional support is a sign of strength and resilience. Whether you're a patient or a caregiver, taking care of your physical, emotional, and practical needs is vital for your well-being and the well-being of your loved one.

9.1 Choosing the Right Healthcare Team

One of the most critical decisions you'll make when facing a cancer diagnosis is selecting the right healthcare team. Your healthcare providers will play a central role in your treatment, support, and overall well-being throughout your cancer journey. In this section, we'll explore essential steps to help you choose a healthcare team that aligns with your needs and preferences.

The Significance of Your Healthcare Team

Your healthcare team will influence various aspects of your cancer experience:

1. **Treatment Plans:** They will design and oversee your treatment plan, which can include surgery, chemotherapy, radiation, immunotherapy, and more.
2. **Support and Guidance:** They will provide medical guidance, emotional support, and resources to help you navigate the complexities of cancer.
3. **Communication:** Effective communication with your healthcare team is vital for understanding your diagnosis, treatment options, and prognosis.

4. **Advocacy:** Your healthcare team should advocate for your best interests and collaborate with you in making informed decisions about your care.

Creating Your Healthcare Team

Primary Healthcare Provider:

o **Choose a Trusted PCP:** Start by selecting a primary care physician (PCP) you trust. Your PCP will serve as a coordinator for your care.

Oncologist:

o **Select an Oncologist:** Seek an oncologist who specializes in your type of cancer. Look for experience, expertise, and a compassionate approach.

Surgeon:

o **Surgical Expertise:** If surgery is part of your treatment plan, choose a surgeon experienced in the specific procedure you need.

Radiation Oncologist:

o **Radiation Therapy:** If radiation therapy is recommended, consult with a radiation oncologist experienced in your type of cancer.

Other Specialists:

o **Consult Specialists:** Depending on your diagnosis, you may need to consult additional specialists, such as a medical oncologist, haematologist, or other experts.

Steps to Choose Your Healthcare Team

Research and Referrals:

o **Ask for Recommendations:** Seek recommendations from your PCP, friends, family, and support groups for healthcare providers with a strong reputation.

Credentials and Experience:

o **Verify Credentials:** Confirm that your healthcare providers are board-certified and have experience treating your specific cancer type.

Consult Multiple Providers:

- o **Seek Second Opinions:** Don't hesitate to consult multiple healthcare providers to gather different perspectives and treatment options.

Communication Style:

- o **Open and Clear Communication:** Choose healthcare providers with a communication style that makes you feel heard and respected.

Treatment Approach:

- o **Treatment Philosophy:** Discuss your treatment philosophy and preferences with potential healthcare providers to ensure alignment.

Support Services:

1. **Inquire About Support Services:** Ask about available support services, such as nurse navigators, social workers, or palliative care teams.

Patient-Centered Care:

o **Prioritize Patient-Centered Care:** Look for healthcare providers who prioritize patient-centered care and involve you in decision-making.

Location and Accessibility:

o **Convenience:** Consider the location and accessibility of your healthcare providers, as this can impact your treatment schedule and logistics.

Trust Your Instincts

Ultimately, trust your instincts when choosing your healthcare team. You should feel confident in their abilities and comfortable discussing your concerns, questions, and goals. Your healthcare team should be partners in your cancer journey, working collaboratively to achieve the best possible outcomes.

Regular Communication

Maintain open and regular communication with your healthcare team:

2. **Ask Questions:** Don't hesitate to ask questions about your diagnosis, treatment options, and potential side effects.

3. **Express Concerns:** Share any concerns or symptoms promptly with your healthcare providers.
4. **Collaborate:** Collaborate with your healthcare team to develop a personalized treatment plan that aligns with your goals and values.

Your Healthcare Advocacy Role

As a patient, you have a vital role in advocating for your health:

1. **Educate Yourself:** Learn about your cancer diagnosis, treatment options, and potential side effects. Knowledge empowers you to make informed decisions.
2. **Seek Second Opinions:** Don't be afraid to seek second opinions to explore different treatment approaches and gain peace of mind.
3. **Follow Your Treatment Plan:** Adhere to your treatment plan and attend regular appointments to monitor progress.
4. **Communicate Openly:** Maintain open communication with your healthcare team and express any concerns or changes in your condition.

Conclusion

Choosing the right healthcare team is a significant step in your cancer journey. By researching, evaluating, and communicating with potential providers, you can assemble a team that not only offers expert medical care but also supports you emotionally and collaborates with you in making informed decisions.

9.2 Asking Questions and Advocating for Yourself

When facing a cancer diagnosis, one of the most empowering steps you can take is to actively ask questions and advocate for yourself. Effective communication and self-advocacy are key to understanding your condition, making informed decisions, and receiving the best possible care. In this section, we'll explore the importance of asking questions and provide guidance on how to advocate for your needs and preferences throughout your cancer journey.

The Power of Asking Questions

Asking questions is a fundamental aspect of your cancer journey:

1. **Understanding:** Questions help you understand your diagnosis, treatment options, and potential side effects.
2. **Empowerment:** By seeking information, you empower yourself to actively participate in your healthcare decisions.
3. **Communication:** Asking questions fosters open and honest communication with your healthcare team.

Preparing for Medical Appointments

1. **Write Down Your Questions:** Before each medical appointment, write down a list of questions or concerns you have. This ensures that you don't forget important topics during your visit.

2. **Bring a Notebook:** Bring a notebook to jot down notes, answers to your questions, and any recommendations or instructions from your healthcare provider.

3. **Prioritize Questions:** Start with the most pressing or essential questions. You may not have time to cover everything in one appointment, so prioritize your concerns.

Types of Questions to Ask

Diagnosis and Treatment:

1. What is my specific diagnosis?
2. What are my treatment options, and what are their pros and cons?
3. How will this treatment plan impact my daily life and activities?
4. Side Effects and Complications:
5. What are the potential side effects of the treatment, and how can they be managed?
6. What should I do if I experience side effects or complications?

Prognosis and Expectations:

1. What is my prognosis, and what can I expect in terms of recovery or long-term outcomes?
2. Are there any milestones or markers to track my progress?

Second Opinions:

o Is it advisable to seek a second opinion about my diagnosis or treatment plan?

Support and Resources:

o Are there support groups, resources, or organizations you recommend for patients with my specific cancer type?

Alternative Treatment Options:

o Are there alternative or complementary therapies that may be beneficial for my condition?

Financial and Insurance:

1. What are the financial implications of my treatment, and what resources or assistance are available?
2. How will my insurance cover the costs of my care?

Advocating for Your Needs

Express Your Preferences:

o **Share Your Values:** Communicate your values and preferences with your healthcare team to ensure that your treatment plan aligns with your goals.

Seek Second Opinions:

o **Don't Hesitate:** If you're unsure about your diagnosis or treatment plan, seek a second opinion from another qualified healthcare provider. It's your right.

Collaborate with Your Healthcare Team:

1. **Be an Active Participant**: Collaborate with your healthcare team to make informed decisions. Your input matters.
2. **Report Changes:** If you experience changes in your condition, side effects, or symptoms, promptly report them to your healthcare provider.

Involve a Trusted Advocate:

o **Supportive Friend or Family Member:** Consider involving a trusted friend or family member in your medical appointments to help ask questions and take notes.

Know Your Rights:

o **Patient Rights:** Familiarize yourself with your patient rights, including your right to informed consent, privacy, and access to your medical records.

Trust Your Instincts

Above all, trust your instincts. If something doesn't feel right or if you have concerns about your care, don't hesitate to voice them. Your healthcare team should listen to your input and address your questions and concerns with respect and compassion.

Conclusion

Asking questions and advocating for yourself are essential components of your cancer journey. By actively seeking information, expressing your preferences, and collaborating with your healthcare team, you can navigate your diagnosis and treatment with confidence and ensure that your care aligns with your goals and values.

9.3 Coping with Hospital Stays

Hospital stays are a common part of the cancer journey, whether it's for surgery, chemotherapy, radiation therapy, or other treatments. Being in the hospital can be challenging both physically and emotionally, but with the right strategies and support, you can make the experience more manageable. In this section, we'll explore tips and techniques to help you cope effectively during hospital stays.

Understanding the Hospital Environment

Hospitals can feel overwhelming, especially during the initial stages of your cancer journey. Understanding the environment and knowing what to expect can help ease some of the anxiety:

1. **Familiarize Yourself:** Take a tour of the hospital if possible or ask for a map. Knowing the layout can reduce confusion and stress.
2. **Supportive Staff:** Hospitals have dedicated staff, including nurses, doctors, and support personnel, who are there to care for you and answer your questions.
3. **Visitor Policies:** Understand the hospital's visitor policies, including visiting hours and any restrictions related to the COVID-19 pandemic.

Personal Comfort and Well-Being

Maintaining your comfort and well-being during a hospital stay is essential:

1. **Comfort Items:** Bring personal comfort items like your Favorite blanket, pillow, or pyjamas to make your hospital room feel more like home.

2. **Entertainment:** Bring books, magazines, or electronic devices for entertainment during downtime.

3. **Stay Connected:** Stay connected with loved ones through phone calls, video chats, or messages to maintain a support network.

Managing Stress and Anxiety

Hospital stays can be stressful, but there are strategies to help manage anxiety:

1. **Breathing Exercises:** Practice deep breathing exercises or mindfulness techniques to calm your mind and reduce anxiety.
2. **Communication:** Share your feelings with your healthcare team or a therapist. They can provide guidance and support.
3. **Distraction:** Engage in activities that distract your mind from worry, such as listening to music, watching movies, or doing puzzles.

Advocating for Yourself

Advocating for your needs and preferences during a hospital stay is crucial:

1. **Ask Questions:** Don't hesitate to ask questions about your treatment plan, medications, or any concerns you may have.
2. **Pain Management:** Communicate your pain levels and any discomfort promptly so that your healthcare team can adjust your pain management plan.
3. **Medication Management:** Keep a record of your medications, including dosages and schedules, to ensure you receive the correct treatment.

Supportive Visitors

Having supportive visitors can make a significant difference:

1. **Visitor List:** Create a list of loved ones who can visit you in the hospital. This social connection can boost your spirits.
2. **Visitor Guidelines:** Share visitor guidelines with your loved ones to ensure a smooth and stress-free experience for everyone.

Nutrition and Hydration

Eating well and staying hydrated can promote healing and overall well-being:

1. **Nutritional Support:** Work with a dietitian to plan your meals based on your dietary preferences and restrictions.
2. **Hydration:** Drink plenty of fluids to stay hydrated, especially if you're undergoing treatments that may cause dehydration.

Mobility and Exercise

Maintaining mobility and gentle exercise, when possible, can prevent muscle weakness and promote circulation:

1. **Mobility:** When allowed, move around your room, or go for short walks in the hospital corridor to stay mobile.
2. **Gentle Exercises:** Perform gentle stretching or range-of-motion exercises to prevent stiffness.

Planning for Discharge

As you prepare for discharge, consider the following:

1. **Discharge Plan:** Work with your healthcare team to develop a comprehensive discharge plan, including any necessary home care or follow-up appointments.
2. **Home Environment:** Ensure that your home environment is safe and comfortable for your return.

Conclusion

Coping with hospital stays during your cancer journey can be challenging, but with the right strategies and support, you can navigate this experience with resilience and positivity. Remember that you have a team of healthcare professionals and loved ones who are there to help you through every step of the way.

9.4 Insurance and Billing Tips

Navigating the financial aspects of cancer care can be daunting, but it's an essential part of your journey. Understanding your insurance coverage, managing medical bills, and seeking financial assistance when needed can help reduce stress and ensure you receive the care you need. In this section, we'll provide valuable tips to help you navigate the complex world of insurance and billing.

Understanding Your Insurance

Review Your Policy: Carefully review your health insurance policy to understand what is covered and any limitations or exclusions related to cancer treatment.

1. **Network Providers:** Whenever possible, choose healthcare providers and facilities that are in-network to maximize coverage and minimize out-of-pocket costs.
2. **Prior Authorization:** If your treatment requires pre-authorization, work closely with your healthcare provider's office to ensure it's obtained to avoid coverage denials.
3. **Appeal Denied Claims:** If your insurance denies a claim, don't hesitate to appeal the decision. Sometimes, errors or misunderstandings can be rectified.

Billing and Medical Expenses

Keep Detailed Records: Maintain organized records of all medical bills, insurance correspondence, and receipts for out-of-pocket expenses.

1. **Verify Bills:** Always verify the accuracy of medical bills. Mistakes can occur, and you don't want to pay for services you didn't receive.

2. **Ask for an Itemized Bill:** Request an itemized bill that breaks down charges for each service or procedure. This can help you identify errors and understand the costs.

3. **Negotiate Costs:** If you're facing high out-of-pocket expenses, don't hesitate to negotiate with healthcare providers or explore options for financial assistance.

4. **Payment Plans:** Many healthcare providers offer flexible payment plans. Inquire about these options to make your bills more manageable.

Financial Assistance and Resources

1. **Social Workers:** Hospital social workers can connect you with financial assistance programs, grants, and resources that can help with medical expenses.

2. **Non-Profit Organizations:** Many non-profit organizations provide financial assistance to cancer patients for treatment-related expenses.

3. **Pharmaceutical Assistance Programs:** Some pharmaceutical companies help programs to help cover the cost of medications.

4. **Government Assistance:** Explore government assistance programs like Medicaid or Medicare if you're eligible.

5. **Patient Advocacy Groups:** Reach out to patient advocacy groups that specialize in your type of cancer. They may provide financial support or guidance.

Communication with Your Healthcare Team

1. **Billing Questions:** Don't hesitate to ask your healthcare team for guidance if you have questions or concerns about medical bills or insurance.

2. **Financial Counsellors:** Hospitals often have financial counsellors who can assist you in understanding your bills and exploring financial assistance options.

Preparing for Financial Challenges

1. **Emergency Fund:** If possible, create an emergency fund or savings account to help cover unexpected medical expenses.
2. **Budgeting:** Develop a budget that accounts for medical costs, daily expenses, and any potential changes in income during treatment.
3. **Insurance Advocate**: Consider working with an insurance advocate or healthcare navigator to help you understand your coverage and navigate the insurance process.

Conclusion

Coping with the financial aspects of cancer care can be challenging, but you are not alone. By understanding your insurance, carefully managing medical bills, and seeking financial assistance when needed, you can alleviate some of the financial stress and focus on your health and well-being.

CHAPTER TEN
LIFE AFTER TREATMENT

10.1 Survivorship and Follow-Up Care

Survivorship is a significant milestone in your cancer journey, marking the transition from active treatment to life beyond cancer. While it's a moment of celebration and relief, it's also a time to focus on your ongoing health and well-being. In this section, we'll explore survivorship, the importance of follow-up care, and how to embrace life after cancer.

Understanding Survivorship

1. **Survivorship Defined:** Survivorship begins the moment you're diagnosed with cancer and continues throughout your life, whether you're in active treatment or considered cancer-free.
2. **Physical and Emotional Healing:** Survivorship involves physical healing from treatment side effects and emotional healing from the impact of cancer.
3. **Embracing Life:** It's an opportunity to embrace life fully, focusing on your health, goals, and the things that bring you joy.

Importance of Follow-Up Care

1. **Regular Check-Ups:** Continue with your regular follow-up appointments, even after treatment ends. These appointments are crucial for monitoring your health.

2. **Health Maintenance:** Follow-up care includes screening for cancer recurrence, managing treatment side effects, and addressing any new health concerns.

3. **Psychological Support:** Emotional and psychological support remains important during survivorship. Seek counselling or support groups if needed.

Post-Treatment Self-Care

1. **Healthy Lifestyle:** Embrace a healthy lifestyle with a balanced diet, regular exercise, and adequate sleep to support your overall well-being.
2. **Mindfulness:** Practice mindfulness and stress reduction techniques to manage anxiety and promote emotional healing.
3. **Cancer Screenings:** Continue to adhere to recommended cancer screenings and tests based on your cancer type and risk factors.
4. **Health Education:** Stay informed about your specific cancer type, treatment history, and potential long-term effects to make informed decisions about your health.

Embracing Life After Cancer

1. **Set Goals:** Define personal goals and aspirations for your post-cancer life. What do you want to achieve or experience?
2. **Reconnect:** Reconnect with your passions and interests that may have taken a back seat during treatment.
3. **Support Network:** Nurture your support network and share your feelings and experiences with loved ones.

4. **Celebrate Milestones:** Celebrate cancer-free milestones and achievements as a reminder of your strength and resilience.

Survivorship Challenges

1. **Fear of Recurrence:** It's common to fear cancer recurrence. Acknowledge these feelings and seek support if they become overwhelming.
2. **Body Image:** Treatment may have altered your body. Embrace self-acceptance and seek professional support if body image issues persist.
3. **Long-Term Effects:** Some cancer treatments may have long-term effects. Discuss potential late effects with your healthcare team and develop strategies to manage them.

Supportive Services

1. **Survivorship Clinics:** Some hospitals offer survivorship clinics that provide specialized care and resources for cancer survivors.
2. **Counselling:** Consider counselling or therapy to address any lingering emotional challenges related to your cancer experience.
3. **Support Groups:** Join cancer survivor support groups to connect with others who share similar experiences and feelings.

Conclusion

Survivorship is a unique and meaningful phase of your cancer journey. Embrace it as an opportunity to focus on your well-being, set new goals, and Savor life's joys. Remember that you are not alone; there is a community of survivors and healthcare professionals ready to support you on your path to a vibrant and fulfilling life after cancer.

10.2 Returning to Work and Normalcy

Returning to work and resuming a sense of normalcy after a cancer diagnosis can be a significant milestone on your journey. It represents a step towards reclaiming your life, independence, and self-esteem. In this section, we'll explore strategies and tips to help you transition back to the workplace and everyday life after cancer treatment.

Assessing Your Readiness

1. **Consult with Your Healthcare Team:** Before returning to work, have an open discussion with your healthcare team to determine if you are physically and emotionally ready.
2. **Gradual Transition:** Consider a gradual return to work, starting with part-time hours or modified duties if possible.
3. **Flexible Schedule:** Explore flexible work arrangements or accommodations that can ease your transition, such as telecommuting or adjusted hours.

Open Communication

1. **Notify Your Employer:** Inform your employer about your cancer diagnosis, treatment plan, and anticipated return date. Open communication is key.

2. **Workplace Support:** Discuss your needs and any necessary workplace adjustments with your employer or HR department.

Emotional and Psychological Support

1. **Self-Care:** Prioritize self-care and stress management techniques as you transition back to work. Continue counselling or therapy if beneficial.
2. **Support Groups:** Join cancer survivor support groups to connect with others who have faced similar challenges and share coping strategies.

Managing Side Effects and Fatigue

1. **Energy Management:** Plan your work tasks and breaks to manage fatigue effectively. Listen to your body and rest when needed.
2. **Medication Schedule:** If you're on medication, ensure you adhere to your medication schedule while at work.

Balancing Work and Health

1. **Pace Yourself:** Avoid overcommitting or taking on too much too soon. Gradually increase your workload as you regain strength.
2. **Self-Advocacy:** Advocate for your health by scheduling medical appointments and treatments around your work schedule when possible.

Colleague and Employer Support

1. **Educate Colleagues:** Educate colleagues about your condition, treatment, and potential side effects to foster understanding and empathy.
2. **Employer Resources:** Inquire about employee assistance programs (EAPs) or workplace resources that may be available to support you.

Legal Protections

1. **Know Your Rights:** Familiarize yourself with legal protections for employees with medical conditions, such as the Family and Medical Leave Act (FMLA) in the United States.
2. **Seek Legal Guidance:** If necessary, seek legal counsel to ensure your rights are protected in the workplace.

Transitioning Back to Normalcy

1. **Reconnect with Hobbies:** Reconnect with hobbies, interests, and social activities that bring you joy outside of work.
2. **Set Realistic Goals:** Set realistic goals and expectations for your post-treatment life, both personally and professionally.
3. **Mindful Self-Care:** Continue to prioritize self-care, mindfulness, and stress management in your daily routine.

Conclusion

Returning to work and normalcy after cancer treatment is a significant accomplishment. It reflects your resilience and determination to embrace life once again. Remember that this transition is a personal journey, and it's okay to seek support and accommodations as needed. You've faced adversity and emerged stronger, and now you could create a fulfilling life beyond cancer.

10.3 Relationship Changes

A cancer diagnosis can have a profound impact on your relationships with loved ones, friends, and even yourself. As you navigate this challenging journey, it's important to recognize and address the changes that may occur in your relationships. In this section, we'll explore strategies and insights to help you navigate these changes with understanding and resilience.

Self-Reflection and Acceptance

1. **Understand Your Feelings:** Acknowledge the emotional changes you may be experiencing and give yourself permission to feel a range of emotions, including anger, sadness, and fear.
2. **Self-Compassion:** Be kind to yourself. Understand that it's okay to have moments of vulnerability and that you don't have to be strong all the time.

Communication Is Key

1. **Open Dialogue:** Foster open and honest communication with your loved ones. Share your thoughts, fears, and needs with them.
2. **Active Listening:** Practice active listening when your loved ones share their concerns and feelings with you. It's a two-way street.

Support from Loved Ones

1. **Lean on Your Support Network:** Allow your loved ones to provide emotional support and assistance when needed. Let them be there for you.
2. **Offer Guidance:** Share resources and information about your cancer type and treatment with your loved ones. Education can ease their fears and help them understand your experience.

Setting Boundaries

1. **Respect Your Limits:** Recognize your physical and emotional limits. It's okay to set boundaries with others when necessary.
2. **Empowerment:** Setting boundaries empowers you to prioritize self-care and your well-being.

Relationship Changes with Spouse or Partner

1. **Intimacy:** Understand that intimacy may change due to physical and emotional factors. Communicate openly with your partner about your needs and concerns.
2. **Seek Support:** Consider couples therapy or counselling to navigate the emotional impact of cancer on your relationship.

Family Dynamics

1. **Family Roles:** Acknowledge that family roles may shift as loved ones take on new responsibilities to support you during treatment.
2. **Family counselling:** Family counselling can help address any conflicts or changes in dynamics that arise.

Friendships

1. **Changing Friendships:** Recognize that some friendships may change or fade during your cancer journey. Focus on nurturing those that provide support and understanding.
2. **New Connections:** Seek out cancer support groups or networks where you can connect with others who understand your experience.

Dealing with Unsupportive Relationships

1. **Choose Your Battles:** Decide when it's worth addressing unsupportive or negative relationships. Sometimes, it's best to distance yourself from toxic influences.
2. **Focus on Positivity:** Surround yourself with positivity and those who uplift and support you.

Professional Help

1. **Therapy or counselling:** Consider individual therapy or counselling to address the emotional toll of relationship changes and seek guidance on coping strategies.
2. **Support Groups:** Join support groups or online communities where you can connect with others who have experienced similar relationship challenges.

Conclusion

Cancer can lead to profound changes in your relationships, but it also offers an opportunity for growth and deeper connections. Embrace open communication, set boundaries, and seek support when needed. Remember that it's okay to ask for help, lean on your support network, and prioritize self-care as you navigate these changes. Your relationships may evolve, but your strength and resilience will shine through.

10.4 Celebrating Milestones

Amid the challenges of a cancer diagnosis and treatment, it's essential to recognize and celebrate the significant milestones you achieve along your journey. These milestones represent your resilience, strength, and determination, and they deserve to be acknowledged and cherished. In this section, we'll explore the importance of celebrating milestones and offer creative ideas to mark these moments with joy and gratitude.

Why Celebrate Milestones

1. **Acknowledge Progress:** Celebrating milestones allows you to acknowledge the progress you've made, both physically and emotionally.
2. **Boost Morale:** Recognizing your achievements can boost your morale and inspire you to keep moving forward.
3. **Share Joy:** Celebrating milestones with loved ones creates moments of joy and brings you closer together.

Types of Milestones

1. **Treatment Milestones:** Mark the completion of treatment phases, such as finishing chemotherapy or radiation.

2. **Health Milestones:** Celebrate improvements in your health, like reaching a specific recovery goal or milestone.

3. **Personal Achievements:** Recognize personal achievements, whether they are related to your cancer journey or unrelated passions and interests.

Creative Ways to Celebrate Milestones

1. **Celebrate with Loved Ones:** Host a small gathering or dinner with family and friends to commemorate your milestone.

2. **Create a Memory Journal:** Keep a milestone journal where you record your thoughts, feelings, and accomplishments.

3. **Symbolic Acts:** Light a candle, release balloons, or plant a tree as symbolic acts of celebration and renewal.

4. **Plan a Special Outing:** Treat yourself to a special outing, whether it's a day at the spa, a picnic in the park, or a visit to a Favorite restaurant.

5. **DIY Art Project:** Engage in a creative art project that reflects your journey and your milestone. Painting, crafting, or writing poetry can be therapeutic.

6. **Share Your Story:** Consider sharing your story with others through writing, speaking, or joining a support group. Your experiences can inspire and empower others.

Gratitude and Reflection

1. **Gratitude Journal:** Start a gratitude journal to reflect on the positive aspects of your journey and the people who have supported you.
2. **Letters of Appreciation:** Write letters of appreciation to those who have been by your side, expressing your gratitude for their support.
3. **Self-Reflection:** Take moments to reflect on your personal growth, resilience, and newfound perspectives.

Setting New Goals

1. **Set New Goals:** After celebrating a milestone, set new goals for yourself, whether they are related to your health, career, or personal interests.
2. **Dream Board:** Create a dream board or vision board that represents your aspirations and goals for the future.

Conclusion

Celebrating milestones on your cancer journey is a way to honour your resilience and embrace the positive moments during adversity. Whether it's completing treatment, achieving a personal goal, or simply finding joy in everyday life, each milestone is a testament to your strength. Share these moments with loved ones, reflect on your journey, and set new goals to continue moving forward with hope and determination.

ACKNOWLEDGMENTS

Writing this book has been a deeply personal and meaningful journey, and I want to take a moment to express my gratitude to the many people who have supported and inspired me along the way.

First and foremost, I want to acknowledge the incredible strength and resilience of all those who have faced a cancer diagnosis. Your courage and determination are a constant source of inspiration.

To the healthcare professionals, doctors, nurses, and support staff who work tirelessly to provide care, guidance, and compassion to cancer patients, your dedication is immeasurable.

I extend my heartfelt thanks to the caregivers, family members, and friends who stand by the side of those battling cancer. Your unwavering support is a testament to the power of love and compassion.

I'm grateful for the countless individuals who shared their personal stories, insights, and tips with me, helping to shape the content of this book. Your experiences have added depth and authenticity to these pages.

I'd like to thank my editor and the publishing team for their guidance, expertise, and dedication to making this book a reality.

To my loved ones, for their patience, encouragement, and understanding during the writing process, you have been my rock.

Lastly, to the readers, I hope this book serves as a source of knowledge, comfort, and inspiration as you navigate your own cancer journey or support someone you care about. Your resilience and strength are awe-inspiring, and I believe in your ability to face any challenge with grace and determination.

CONCLUSION

As we reach the final page of this book, I want to leave you with a heartfelt message of hope, resilience, and empowerment.

Your journey with cancer, whether you're the patient or a supporting loved one, is a path filled with challenges, uncertainties, and moments of strength you may never have imagined. It's a journey that tests your limits and reveals your incredible capacity for courage.

Throughout this book, we've explored 101 tips and insights to help you navigate the complexities of life with cancer. From understanding your diagnosis and treatment options to coping with emotions, relationships, and everyday life, you've gained a wealth of knowledge and practical advice.

But remember, knowledge alone is not enough. It's the application of that knowledge, combined with your spirit, determination, and the support of your loved ones, that will guide you through the darkest days and lead you toward the brighter ones.

Cancer is a formidable adversary, but you are stronger than you know. You have within you the power to face each day with courage and resilience. You have the capacity to find joy in the smallest of moments, to cherish the love that surrounds you, and to make decisions that align with your values and priorities.

Your journey is unique, and there is no one-size-fits-all approach to living with cancer. You are the author of your story, and you could shape it in a way that reflects your strength, your dreams, and your hopes for the future.

As you move forward, remember that you are not alone. There is a community of individuals who have walked a similar path, who understand the ups and downs, and who are ready to offer support and encouragement when you need it most.

In the face of adversity, you've shown resilience. Amid uncertainty, you've discovered courage. And in the presence of love and support, you've found the strength to continue the journey.

May your path be filled with moments of healing, joy, and triumph. May your spirit remain unbreakable, and may your life be a testament to the power of the human spirit.